Pregnant
women with drug history

Tara K. Lawler

Acknowledgements

I would like to express my gratitude to all the women who generously gave up their time to tell their stories. This research would not be possible without them, and I was so very appreciative of the time that they gave freely to me. Their candid recounts of their lives and experiences will never be forgotten. In addition, I would like to express my thanks to all the dedicated and passionate health care and social care providers and the DCJ workers who took time out of their busy schedules to speak with me- thank you.

I would like to thank my supervisors Professor Angela Dawson, Emeritus Professor Cathrine Fowler and Associate Professor Stephanie Taplin for their generous support, encouragement and supervision through this process. Your attention to detail, your knowledge and incredibly fast feedback has been very much appreciated. Additionally, your belief in me, even when I doubted myself has been unwavering.

I would like to acknowledge my children who have grown from young children to teenagers while I embarked on this PhD journey. As a single parent, this has been hard on all of us at times. Especially during COVID-19. As a frontline health care worker, I was required to undertake extra work as part of the pandemic response team in the South Eastern Sydney Local Health District. This coupled with supervising my children who were (attempting) to engage with home schooling meant that I needed to extend my candidature. I am so grateful for the support that the UTS Graduate Research School provided to me. Thank you, Monty and Millie, for being so understanding and I look forward to spending more time with both of you.

Ultimately though, I hope that this research does justice for the all the women and their care providers who were interviewed. My overall vision is a health and social care system that is more flexible, compassionate and responsive to these women and their children's needs. I truly believe that as a society we will strive for and achieve better outcomes for some of our most vulnerable.

Abbreviations

ACT: Australian Capital Territory
AOD: Alcohol and other drug
ATS: Amphetamine type substances
AVO: Apprehended violence order
BBVI: Blood-borne viral infectious
BCAP: Brief Child Abuse Potential
BZD: Benzodiazepines
CMA: Crystal methamphetamine ('ice')
DOCS: Department of Community Services (now DCJ)
DCJ: Department of Communities and Justice (formally FACS, and DOCS)
EDPS: Edinburgh Postnatal Depression Scale
ETOH: Ethyl alcohol
FACS: Family and Community Services (now DCJ)
FDTC: Family Drug Treatment Court
HCV: Hepatitis C virus
HIV: Human immunodeficiency virus
IDU: Injecting drug users
IPV: Intimate partner violence
KPCS: Karitane Parenting Confidence Scale
KRC: Kirketon Road Centre
LARC: Long-acting reversible contraception
LSNS: Lubben Social Network Scale
NAS: Neonatal abstinence syndrome
NDS: National Drug Strategy
NGO: Non-government organisation
NSW: New South Wales
OAT: Opiate agonist treatment (such as methadone or buprenorphine)
OOHC: Out of home care
OUD: Opioid use disorder
PFC: Pregnancy family conferences
PHC: Primary health care
PSE: Parenting self efficacy
PWID: People who inject drugs
SDM: Structured Decision Making
SRH: Sexual and reproductive health
STI: Sexually transmitted infection
SUD: Substance use disorder
THC: Tetrahydrocannabinol
USA: United States of America

Glossary

Aboriginal: A person of Aboriginal or/and Torres Strait Islander decent

Addiction: An inability to stop doing or using something, especially something harmful

Current or recent injecting drug user: A person who has injected drugs in the previous six months

Harm minimisation: Building safe, healthy and resilient communities through preventing, responding and reducing alcohol, tobacco and other drugs related health, social and economic harms. This includes harm reduction, supply reduction and demand reduction.

Harm reduction: Refers to policies, programmes and practices that aim to minimise negative health, social and legal impacts associated with drug use, drug policies and drug laws.

New mothers: This includes women who have a new baby. They may also have other children

Perinatal period: Pregnancy and the first year postpartum

Reunification: Placement of a child back into care with their birth mother

Substance use disorder: The impact of addiction on a person's brain and behaviour, leading to a person's inability to control their use of substances

Substantiated case (child protection): When the professional opinion of officers of the child protection authority, is that there is reasonable cause to believe that a child has been, is being, or is likely to be abused, neglected or otherwise harmed.

Style notes

'Single quotation marks' with *italics* are verbatim quotes, phrases or words from individual study participants (women, health and social care providers and Department of Community and Justice workers).

"Double quotation marks" with *italics* are verbatim quotes of study participants when describing a quote from a different person

Main quotes are indented within paragraphs and assigned single quotation marks. For quotes over three lines, there are no quotation marks. All quotes are italicised.

At the end of each indented quote a pseudonym and interview number was assigned.

Explanatory inserts within quotes are bracketed and not italicised.

Table of contents

List of Tables

List of Diagrams

Abstract

Background: Maternal substance use disorders are considered a significant public health issue in Australia and globally. While it does not necessarily lead to inadequate parenting, it is strongly linked to poorer health and social outcomes for their infants. Women with substance use disorders have unique experiences compared to men, including complex histories, mental health disorders and trauma from intimate partner violence. Additionally, it is estimated that many of these women have children, and approximately 60-70% of Australian children were removed from households where substance abuse was present. Women who inject drugs face multiple challenges and are some of the most vulnerable women in society. Yet, there is a dearth of literature in Australia and internationally that describes these women's needs, experiences and preferences for care.

Aim: This study aimed to determine the health and psychosocial needs and experiences of pregnant women and women who have recently given birth and are recent or current injecting drug users in NSW, Australia. It explored experiences of accessing care and examine how service providers can best support, plan and deliver appropriate evidence-based care to meet the needs of these women.

Methods: This study employed a mixed-methods exploratory case study design. This included a situational analysis, a guideline review, quantitative instruments and a series of qualitative interviews. Thirteen women, 13 health and social care providers and six Department of Community and Justice workers participated in interviews

Findings: This is the first known Australian study that identifies the health care experiences and needs of pregnant women and new mothers who are current injecting drug users. Findings indicate these women have multiple unmet health and psychosocial needs, and at times health and social care systems are not providing the required care. Women interacted with systems that held power over them, failed to recognise their strengths and for some women, basic needs such as housing were not met. The complexities within these women's lives including intimate partner violence, mental health, trauma, and substance use meant stability was difficult to achieve.

Conclusion: Policies, guidelines and a one-stop-shop model of integrated primary health care that holistically meets the needs of women has the potential to break the cycle of adversity by addressing multiple layers of health and psychosocial issues. A trial of models of care that proactively targets women with substance use disorders in their pregnancy and beyond such as nurse-led models of care and a Sustained Home Visiting Program are urgently required. Change is possible, but committed action is essential.

CHAPTER ONE: BACKGROUND

Summary, Background and Origins of Research

Women with substance use disorders (SUDs) have unique experiences compared to men. While more men than women use drugs, there is evidence that overall levels of SUDs in women are increasing. Additionally, women with SUDs often have complex histories, including mental health disorders such as depression and anxiety and trauma from intimate partner violence (IPV). For pregnant women and women with children, these issues are further complicated. Furthermore, their infants and children are at risk of a range of adverse outcomes that can continue through to adulthood. Positively, SUD treatment can ameliorate some of the adverse outcomes for women, their infants and children yet, women are less likely to access SUD treatment than men (Grella et al., 2006, Grella et al., 2009, Ashley et al., 2003).

Substance use disorders (SUDs) are complex and multifactorial chronic conditions that are preventable and treatable (McLellan et al., 2014 p.69, Street et al., 2004). Women with SUDs face many medical and social problems, including hepatitis C (HCV), mental health disorders and homelessness (Haber and Day, 2014). In addition, these women experience stigma, including from health care workers (Brener et al., 2007a). Babies born to mothers with SUDs are at greater risk of co-morbidities and perinatal complications when compared to mothers without a SUD (Miles et al., 2010b). Notably, newborns are at risk of neonatal abstinence syndrome (NAS) which occurs when a mother uses opiates during pregnancy (Finnegan and Kaltenbach, 1992). Even though NAS is related to maternal opiate use, opioid replacement therapy such as methadone or buprenorphine is the standard of care for opioid dependency during pregnancy (Jones et al., 2006, Finnegan, 1991). This treatment leads to improved obstetric and neonatal outcomes (Jones et al., 2014).

Maternal substance use disorders are considered a significant public health problem in Australia and globally (Forray, 2016). While it does not necessarily lead to inadequate parenting (Street et al., 2004) it is strongly linked to child abuse and neglect (McGlade et al., 2009, Prindle et al., 2018, Tsantefski et al., 2014), and poor childhood developmental outcomes (Abdel-Latif et al., 2007). Additionally, substance abuse is commonly cited as a factor related to a child being placed in out-of-home care (OOHC) (McGlade et al., 2009, Prindle et al., 2018).

In Australia's most populous state of New South Wales (NSW), children and adolescents up to the age of 18 who cannot live with their birth families are provided with OOHC. As of 30 June 2020, approximately 46,000 children were living in OOHC, equating to approximately 8 per 1,000 children. Between 30 June 2017 and 30 June 2020, the number of children in OOHC rose by 7% (from 43,100 to 46,000). However, promisingly the rate of children in out-of-home was relatively stable (AIHW, 2021a). Concerningly though, is the rate of Australian Aboriginal and Torres Strait Islander, named hereafter Aboriginal, children in OOHC, where the rate was 59.4 per 1,000 children (AIHW, 2019). This rate of OOHC is ten times that of non-Aboriginal children (AIHW, 2019) and has drawn comparisons with the 'stolen generation' which is a dark part of Australian history where Aboriginal children were forcibly removed from their birth families by the Australian federal and state government agencies and church missions (O'Donnell et al., 2019). This policy pervaded the lives of Aboriginal Australian's from the early 1900s and continued through to the 1970s, and the legacy of this trauma continues to negatively impact the health and wellbeing of Aboriginal communities (O'Donnell et al., 2019).

Estimates suggest that approximately 60-70% of Australian children taken into OOHC were removed from households where substance abuse was present (Fernandez and Lee, 2013). While there is support and care for mothers who use substances during pregnancy, there is a scarcity of research examining how women perceive the support provided to them during this vulnerable time; and their health and psychosocial needs. Therefore, this study aimed to highlight the health and psychosocial needs and experiences of women during the perinatal period who have a history of recent or current injecting drug use (IDU). Injecting drug use poses unique risks and challenges and therefore necessitates particular attention. For this study, the perinatal period is defined as during pregnancy and the first year postpartum (Garcia and Yim, 2017).

Overview of substance use disorders and patterns of use

A definition of substance use disorders

A substance is defined as a compound that can alter one's senses and cause health and social problems (McLellan, 2017). These substances may be legal such as tobacco and alcohol, or illegal, such as heroin and cocaine and can also include controlled pharmaceuticals such as morphine (McLellan, 2017). Addiction to a substance is defined as a chronic and relapsing disorder that can result in long-lasting changes to the brain, including, compulsive drug seeking and continued use, even though there are negative consequences (NIDA, 2020).

Addiction is now recognised as a chronic brain disease with physiological and molecular changes that occur after repeated drug exposures and persist for a long time after drug discontinuation (Volkow and Li, 2005). This view of a chronic brain disease is contentious in that it identifies addiction as deterministic and it fails to account for heterogeneity in remission and recovery, and emphasises a compulsive dimension of addiction (Heilig et al., 2021). However, ignoring this model can increase stigma and hamper efforts to find effective solutions through a systematic understanding of the underlying phenomena (Heilig et al., 2021).

The term SUD describes the addiction's impact on an individual's overall functioning and can be defined as mild, moderate or severe according to the level of impairment (Volkow and Li, 2005). These impairments may be health problems, disability or failure to meet primary responsibilities at work, school, or home (SAMHSA, 2014). A diagnosis of SUD is based on evidence of impaired control, social impairment, risky use, and pharmacological criteria and are determined by the number of diagnostic criteria met by an individual, such as hazardous use, higher tolerance, and physical and psychological problems associated with use (American Psychiatric Association, 2013). A SUD varies from substance misuse which is the use of substances at high doses or in inappropriate situations that can cause a health or social problem. An example is binge drinking by an individual that leads embarrassment and/or risk taking such as unprotected sexual intercourse (McLellan, 2017).

It is now understood that 40-60% of the vulnerabilities to addiction can be attributed genetically (Volkow and Li, 2005). Environmental influences also play a significant role in availability, concurrent mental illness, and other social and economic issues, including parental drug use. The presence of parental SUD is associated with the development of a SUD in their children (Volkow and Li, 2005). However, the effect on the child can be reduced if the parent receives treatment (Arria et al., 2012).

The patterns of substance use
Many people experiment with a drug or drugs at some point in their lifetime, evident by the increasing levels of drug use worldwide. In 2019 around 269 million people were reported to use drugs, and these figures have increased by 30% compared to 2009 (UNDOC, 2020). Whilst some people may become frequent users, a subset will develop an ongoing or chronic SUD (Hser et al., 2007).

Drug use trends in Australia are monitored by The National Drug Strategy Survey Household Report which is the leading survey of licit and illicit drug use and drug trends. In 2019, this survey found that 43% of Australians aged 14 or over had ever used an illicit drug in their lifetime and 16.4% within the preceding 12 months (NDSHS, 2019). These figures, although relatively stable, have increased. For example, in 2016, 38% of Australians aged 14 or over had used an illicit drug, and 13.4% within the preceding 12 months (NDSHS, 2019).

In Australia, the most common illicit drugs used in the previous 12 months of 2019 were cannabis (11.6%), followed by cocaine (4.2%) and ecstasy (3.0%). These numbers again increased between 2016 to 2019. With cannabis use up from 10.4%, cocaine from 2.5% and ecstasy up from 2.2% (AIHW, 2020a). Positively, the use of pharmaceutical drugs for non-medical purposes has declined from 4.8% in 2016 to 4.2% in 2019 (AIHW, 2020a). This reduction may be due to policy reforms regarding access to prescription and over the counter medicines (TGA, 2019).

Injecting drug use, which is related to multiple harms, fluctuated in the Australian population between 2001 and 2019, from a low of 0.3% in 2013 and 2019 to a high of 0.6% in 2001 (AIHW, 2020a). However, recent use of heroin has remained stable at about 0.1% (AIHW, 2020a). Although heroin use is low, the frequency is much higher than other drugs, with 49% of users using heroin as often as weekly. Among people who inject drugs (PWID) in general, 41% inject twice a week or more (AIHW, 2017a), which signifies a greater propensity for injecting drug use-related harm. Among those who injected any drug, 78% reported using any form of methamphetamine in the previous six months (AIHW, 2020a). While the use of methamphetamines or amphetamine type substances (ATS) has declined from 2.1 to 1.3% from 2013 to 2019, methamphetamine use, commonly known as 'ice', is increasing, and most methamphetamine users stated that 'ice' was their primary drug in 2016 (AIHW, 2020a).

Definition of recent and current injecting drug use

Addiction is a relapsing condition, and consequently it is difficult to determine a cut-off to define permanent versus short-term cessation of IDU (and therefore 'current'/'recent' versus 'former' PWID) (Larney et al., 2015). Additionally, varying definitions are used in the literature to define current and or recent IDU with definitions ranging from one month to one year (EMCDDA, 2010, WHO, 2012). For the purpose of this study, any woman who has had at least one episode of IDU within the last six months is defined as a recent or current PWID.

Policy response to substance use

Harm reduction is increasingly seen as the predominant policy in addressing substance use in the Western world (Des Jarlais, 2017). Challenges along the way, such as the 'War on Drugs', introduced in 1971 by President Nixon, and the 'Just Say No' campaign of the 1980s, have hampered harm reduction efforts (Reynolds, 2020). However, harm reduction policy is now a consensus more than a controversy throughout Europe, the United States of America (USA) and Australia (Miovský et al., 2020). Even in the USA, where there are varying harm reduction policies across the different states, the support for pragmatism in response to substance use is the predominant view, given the rise of the opioid crisis (Nadelmann and LaSalle, 2017).

In Australia, the policy response to drug and alcohol problems was shaped by the human immunodeficiency virus (HIV) crisis in the mid-1980s. Before this, alcohol and drug problems were afforded little attention (DoH, 2004). In 1985, the Australian National Drug Strategy (NDS) was launched, and one of its key elements was to prevent an epidemic of HIV transmitted through IDU (DoH, 2004). The NDS, which has been around for over 35 years and essentially has bipartisan political support (Lancaster and Ritter, 2014), is a guiding document for the development of legislation, policy, and practice around drug and alcohol issues, with its fundamental underlying principle being harm minimisation (Haber and Day, 2014). Examples of harm minimisation programs for PWID include: needle and syringe programs, pharmacotherapy, rehabilitation programs, counselling, and medically supervised injecting facilities (Harm Reduction International, 2021).

Treatment of substance use disorders

Treatment of SUDs has classically been reactive and has focused on acute interventions instead of being managed as a chronic and relapsing condition (Tai and Volkow, 2013). People with a SUD can present with similar patterns to many other types of chronic illness such as diabetes type II and hypertension in terms of onset, and require regular support and monitoring to prevent relapse (McLellan et al., 2000). Stability and reduction or cessation of drug use is possible when the person engages with effective treatment, and there are strong linkages with and between systems of care (Saitz et al., 2008).

In Australia, there is a whole-of-government strategic approach to managing drug and alcohol issues which is funded by both the states and the Federal Government (Haber and Day, 2014). Typically, the states manage substance use treatment programs such as opiate treatment services and counselling which are delivered through a mix of public and not-for-profit organisations. There are also a small number of private treatment programs (Haber and Day, 2014). Publicly funded drug and alcohol treatment programs such as opiate treatment services and case management are often attached to hospitals or near a hospital campus. These are managed by addiction medicine specialists and include other professional staff such as nurses, counsellors and social workers (Haber and Day, 2014).

The non-government sector provides a wide range of specialist prevention and treatment services throughout NSW, including opiate agonist treatment (OAT), such as methadone, buprenorphine, counselling, case management, withdrawal management, and residential and day rehabilitation programs (NSW Health, 2017b). Costs for treatment vary, but these usually include a payment from a person's fortnightly government-provided welfare payment and are supported through the Government's national health insurance system, Medicare.

Covid 19 has impacted SUD service delivery and access to treatment. Providers have had to change modes of treatment delivery, including decreasing bed capacity at residential rehabilitation and withdrawal services, reducing the intake of new clients and the introduction of telehealth (Deacon et al., 2020). Unfortunately, this has also meant that group sessions were cancelled or moved to telehealth forums, prescription review periods increased for medications such as methadone, there have been increased wait times, and some centres have closed (DoH, 2020). Because of these service delivery changes and during the pandemic, it is likely that there are further adverse outcomes for people with substance use disorders. People with SUD are already marginalised and stigmatised and are known to have poor access to health services in the first place, and Covid-19 could lead to further long term issues (Deacon et al., 2020).

Outcomes of People Who Inject Drugs

People who inject drugs warrant particular attention. Injecting drug use is of major public health concern, and it is widely documented in the literature that PWID are at risk of increases morbidity, mortality and a range of social problems. For examples, see: (Brener et al., 2007b, Meyers et al., 2021, Haber and Day, 2014, Mathers et al., 2013). The following section will describe outcomes for PWID for the following: physical health, sexual and reproductive health, and mental and social health outcomes.

Health and medical outcomes

People who inject drugs experience multiple adverse health consequences, including a higher risk of death from overdose (Mathers et al., 2013), osteomyelitis, pneumonia (Cornford and Close 2016), endocarditis and have increased hospitalisation rates (Haber and Day, 2014). Deep vein thrombosis is also common due to ongoing injecting and poor venous access and consequences of this can more serious outcomes such as pulmonary emboli and even death (Cooke and Fletcher, 2006).

In addition, PWID are disproportionately affected by blood-borne viral infectious (BBVI), including HIV, hepatitis B (HBV) and hepatitis C (HCV) (Zimmermann et al., 2019). Estimates suggest that 2.8 million people who inject worldwide live with HIV, 1.4 million have chronic hepatitis B and 8.2 million have HCV (Degenhardt et al., 2017). Due to the Covid-19 pandemic, there have been delays in releasing HCV surveillance reports; however, the most recent Australian report estimated that in 2017, approximately 170,000 people in Australia had chronic HCV, with approximately 80% of these infections acquired through IDU (Burnet Institute and Kirby Institute, 2019). Positively there has been an 8% decrease in new notifications from 2015 to 2018 and a 51% reduction in hepatitis C RNA prevalence in this same period (Burnet Institute and Kirby Institute, 2019). Chronic HCV can reduce quality of life (Rodger et al., 1999) and lead to serious complications such as liver cirrhosis and cancer (Alter and Seeff, 2000). In 2015, just under one third (30.6%) of people with HCV were female (The Kirby Institute, 2016).

Concerningly, overdose due to drug use is on the rise in Australia and there has been an increase in the number of people who die from unintentional overdose (Pennington Institute, 2020). Overdose is primarily from a combination of prescribed opiates and benzodiazepine (BZD), which are injected in addition to heroin. In 2019 there were 2070 drug-induced deaths, and 1556 of these were unintentional (Pennington Institute, 2020). These figures highlight the need for effective and urgent public health action. One public health initiative to address this issue is naloxone which reverses the effect of opioids (Miller et al., 2022). Given its life saving potential the Australian Government has invested $3.9 million towards funding a Take Home Naloxone Pilot project. Under the pilot, naloxone is available free to people who may either experience, or witness, an opioid overdose. No prescription is required (DoH, 2022). Despite the clear benefits of Naloxone, unfortunately varying uptake across different jurisdiction and lack of timely roll out in prisons have hampered implementation of this program in Australia (Dietze et al., 2020).

Sexual and reproductive health outcomes
Women who inject drugs are at higher risk for sexually transmitted infections (STIs) such as chlamydia and gonorrhoea. These infections may be due to multiple partners, low use of condoms, and sex work (Khan et al., 2013). These women are also twice as likely to have unintended pregnancies and birth complications. For example, a Sydney-based study focused on women with a history of IDU and who were on OAT reported a higher average number of births, pregnancies, and stillborn babies than the Australian population (Black et al., 2012b). In this study of 302 women, nearly eight out of ten pregnancies were reported as unintended. These rates are at least twice that of women who do not inject drugs (Taft et al., 2018).

Other studies of women who inject drugs have reported similar outcomes, where many pregnancies came as a surprise (Cleveland et al., 2016, Terplan et al., 2015). In these studies, women experienced complications in previous pregnancies, including prematurity. However, despite these challenges, the women saw the current pregnancy as an opportunity to change (Cleveland et al., 2016, Terplan et al., 2015).

Contraceptive use for women with SUDs has been found to be low compared to other populations of women. In a systematic review of 21 papers exploring contraception use in women with SUDs, Terplan et al. (2015) found that women with SUDs used contraception 56% of the time versus 81% of non-drug-using comparison populations. This illustrates the need for maternal and reproductive health care and counselling amongst this group of women and care that considers the wide range of social and medical complications and harms associated with IDU.

Mental health and women with SUDs

Women with SUDs are more likely to be diagnosed with mental health problems than women without SUDs. For example, one Australian study of 170 women on OAT treatment found that 54.2% had been recently diagnosed with a psychiatric illness (Taplin and Mattick, 2013). These results are consistent with overseas studies. For example, a study from the USA found that of 396 mothers with SUDs, 46% had comorbid mental disorders, with more than half having two or more mental disorder diagnoses (Hser et al., 2015). Poor mental health in women is often associated with adverse events in early life and can severely impact their wellbeing, and contributes to poorer outcomes for their babies and children (NDARC, 2015). Critically, the development of infant-parent attachment can be affected in this cohort of mothers (Suchman et al., 2006).

Social and financial issues

People who inject drugs face multiple social issues. In addition, they are often marginalised and stigmatised by society, including health care workers (Brener et al., 2007b, Meyers et al., 2021). Stigma negatively affects people with SUD related issues, affecting SUD treatment uptake and completion (Brener et al., 2010) and impacts mental and physical health (Ahern et al., 2007). Furthermore, women with SUDs and mothers are stigmatised more so than men as it goes against the ideals of femininity and being a nurturer and carer (Lee and Boeri, 2017).

Moreover, SUDs are associated with increased social isolation, debt, stress and illness, and even early death. Socioeconomic status and substance use can be bidirectional, where economic status can be related to drug use and vice versa, demonstrating the cyclical nature of substance use and its outcomes (Spooner and Hetherington, 2005). Poverty is related to stress, poor health, poor literacy and poor mental health and low socioeconomic status communities are often marked by high unemployment, drug use and crime. These issues provide a cultural environment conducive to problematic drug use and can profoundly impact children living in these environments, and these impacts can last a lifetime (Spooner and Hetherington, 2005).

Many studies have found that high levels of IPV are present in relationships that involve substance use (Schumm et al., 2018, Ferrari et al., 2014, Rosenberg, 2011, Macy and Goodbourn, 2012). For example, an Australian study found that 18% of 170 women with a SUD had recently taken out an apprehended violence order in response to IPV (Taplin and Mattick, 2011). However, no single factor can explain the reasons for the high levels of violence, but it may be an interplay between substance use, the context of intoxication, withdrawal and addiction, and wider dynamics of power and control and other psychological vulnerabilities (Gilchrist et al., 2019). These high rates of IPV highlight the need for urgent evidence-based interventions to counteract some of the adverse outcomes associated with IPV, including higher rates of children removed into care (Tsantefski et al., 2014).

Mothers and Substance Use Disorders

Substance use disorders and effects on women and children

Women with SUD warrant particular attention as they are most likely to be the primary carers for children when substance use is present in a household (Douglas and Walsh, 2010, Taplin and Mattick, 2011). However, it is difficult to estimate the proportion of households where substance use is present, as these questions are not routinely asked in population-based surveys. One study from 2016 that reported on this matter found that 14% of adults with a child aged 0 – 14 used an illicit substance within the 12 months before being surveyed (AIHW, 2020c).

Substance use in pregnancy presents unique challenges. Many mothers cease drug use during pregnancy (Hayatbakhsh et al., 2011), however a small proportion of mothers continue to use drugs at levels that are harmful to the mother and the developing foetus. While it is challenging to ascertain how many mothers continue to use drugs in pregnancy, one study conducted in 2004 found that of all pregnancies in public hospitals in NSW and the Australian Capital Territory (ACT), 879 were born to illicit drug-using mothers during a 12-month period. This is a prevalence rate of 1.4% (Abdel-Latif et al., 2013).

Babies born to mothers who use drugs during pregnancy have higher morbidities and perinatal complications than mothers who do not use drugs during pregnancy (Miles et al., 2010a). These issues include a smaller head circumference, prematurity and perinatal complications such as antenatal haemorrhage and chorioamnionitis (Abdel-Latif et al., 2007). Furthermore, a link has been found between insecure infant-mother attachment for mothers with SUD (Schindler, 2019). As young children, poor levels of cognition, behavioural problems and developmental delays can occur, and these may not be remedied with time (Nygaard et al., 2015).

Neonatal abstinence syndrome is one well-documented outcome of mothers who use opiates during pregnancy. However, OAT, methadone, or buprenorphine as synthetic opiates is the treatment in mothers addicted to heroin and other opiates. Compared to withdrawal or no OAT, OAT is related to a decrease in adverse outcomes (Jones et al., 2008b), and can assist in relapse prevention and limit stress on the unborn foetus. Daily or regular dosing also means that regular engagement with health care providers is required to provide opportunities for treatment and ongoing support (Jones et al., 2008a).

Foetal exposure to drug use can lead to considerable adverse perinatal and childhood outcomes (Abdel-Latif et al., 2013), In addition, SUD is associated with a complex milieu of social determinants such as poverty, low levels of educational attainment, IPV and poor nutrition. Therefore, substance use in pregnancy and its related factors must be identified as early as possible. Universal screening for substance use and misuse is recommended and should occur in all pregnant women to provide support as early as possible (WHO, 2014).

Unfortunately, some women with SUDs approach antenatal care late in their pregnancy or not at all (Burns et al., 2006, Stone, 2015), removing the opportunity for timely antenatal care. Late or lack of engagement in health care during pregnancy can occur for several reasons, including a lack of awareness of their pregnancy (Hepburn, 2004), limited trust in health care services and child protection agencies. In addition, previous negative interactions with health services, feelings of shame, and practical issues, such as having money for transport services to attend appointments, can contribute to a lack of engagement (Stone, 2015). Additionally, guilt for using substances in the first place can mean women do not attend appointments, or if they do attend and have a negative experience, this can compel them to increase their drug use (Roberts and Pies, 2011). As a result, they may withdraw from services (Roberts and Pies, 2011). Stigma free and supportive service delivery can mitigate issues associated with guilt (Roberts and Pies, 2011).

Child protection and harms associated with substance use disorders
In Australia, increasing numbers of children are reported to child protection authorities. Reports occur for a range of reasons such as emotional abuse (52%), neglect (22%), physical abuse (14%),

and sexual abuse (9%), the latter being more common amongst girls (13%) compared to boys (6%) (AIHW, 2021a). The placement of children into OOHC is also rising. Between 30 June 2017 and 30 June 2020 there was a 7% increase in the number of children placed into OOHC (from 43,100 to 46,000). However, during this time, the rate of children in out-of-home was relatively steady at 8 per 1,000 children (AIHW, 2021a).

Children younger than one are more likely to be a confirmed substantiated case or taken into OOHC (AIHW, 2019). As mentioned previously there are disparate rates of Aboriginal children living in OOHC compared to non-Aboriginal children. These high rates of OOHC for Aboriginal children urgently requires attention to prevent further generations from experiencing transgenerational trauma. Practices that support family empowerment, early intervention to address trauma, mental health and substance use, and the delivery of culturally safe practices are interventions that can support positive outcomes for children at risk (O'Donnell et al., 2019).

Substance use on its own is a risk factor for child removal. One Australian study of 171 mothers on methadone found that 42% of these mothers had a child removed and taken into OOHC at birth (Taplin and Mattick, 2013). This study, which focused on women who had a history of IDU (all of whom had at least one child under 16 years of age), found that just over one-third of mothers had current involvement with the child protection system. Thirty-two per cent of these mothers had at least one child in OOHC at the time of the interview. Nearly half had their children removed immediately or within weeks of birth. Internationally, removal rates where substance use is present have been as high as 80% (Schaeffer et al., 2013).

However, it must be recognised that substance use can be a part of many other contributing factors to child removal. Studies that have examined characteristics of women with a history of child protection involvement and SUDs report that these women are mostly financially impoverished, struggling to meet basic needs, coping with trauma, IPV and are mainly unemployed (Marcenko et al., 2011, Tsantefski et al., 2014, Taplin and Mattick, 2013). These findings demonstrate the urgent need for evidence-based and improved interventions to support these vulnerable women and their families (Marmot and Wilkinson, 2003). Interventions such as SUD treatments, including OAT and rehabilitation, have been demonstrated to lessen child protection involvement for mothers with SUDs (McGlade et al., 2009).

Child protection legislation

Australia has a legislative framework regarding the mandatory reporting of at-risk children (AIFS, 2020). Mandatory reporters are required by law to report any instance of actual or suspected child abuse and neglect, including health care professionals, teachers, childcare educators and disability workers (DCJ, 2017a). In addition, and although not mandatory, professionals can also make a prenatal report, which allows for early intervention for pregnant women. One of the aims here is to reduce the likelihood that the child will need to be placed in OOHC (DCJ, 2017a). If an infant or child has been reported and is deemed 'at-risk', they are allocated a caseworker through the NSW Department of Communities and Justice (DCJ). The role of these caseworkers, who are child protection workers, is to support vulnerable families and improve overall outcomes for children and their families (AIFS, 2020). When it is appropriate and case plan goals are met, the case may be closed. When possible, this decision should be made with the family, child, and relevant organisations (DCJ, 2020a).

The Department of Communities and Justice is the leading NSW Government agency responsible for child protection, supporting everyone's right to access justice, and providing help for families by promoting early intervention and inclusion to benefit the whole community (DCJ, 2022). Department of Communities and Justice will be referred to as DCJ in this thesis, and the people employed by them will be referred to as DCJ workers.

Family preservation is the main driver behind the NSW DCJ policy, which operates under an evidenced-based model to keep children with their families, where possible, and it is safe (DCJ, 2021a). Families at risk may be asked to undertake family group conferencing, a strengths-based program that supports families to remain together (DCJ, 2021a). Additionally, if necessary, a court may place a parent under a parenting contract that encourages parents to set goals and accept greater responsibility for the care of their child. This contract may include SUD treatment (DCJ, 2021a). These parental contracts are in place for up to 12 months to allow a parent to attest their ability to parent their infant or child. If this is not possible, permanency outside the home is the aim.

Critics of the legislation have stated that 12 months is an arbitrary period and these timeframes fail to acknowledge the time it takes to recover from trauma and chronic conditions such as SUDs (WLSNSW, 2021). Furthermore, a scoping review by the Australian Institute of Family Studies found no recent empirical data on time to permanency and its impact on child health, wellbeing, or life outcomes (Goldsworthy and Muir, 2019). Rather, the research focuses on factors associated with time to permanency rather than on whether this timing produced better or worse outcomes for the child. Factors that influence the timing to permanency include a child's circumstances, such as if they have a disability, the capacity of the system to plan for permanency effectively, finding suitable carers, and the ability to support biological parents (Goldsworthy and Muir, 2019). Furthermore, while OOHC is an essential part of child protection (Maclean et al., 2016) there are mixed results for some children who enter OOHC, with some studies finding little difference or worsening outcomes for children who have been placed in OOHC (Maclean et al., 2016).

Child and family reunification literature and out of home care
Within the child welfare context, reunification is defined as a process of services provided to families who have a child placed in OOHC, with the intention of returning the child to their families of origin (Carnochan et al., 2013, Delfabbro et al., 2009). Where this is not possible, children are placed into alternative care such as kinship or adoption (Carnochan et al., 2013, Maluccio, 1996).

Where substance use is present in the household, and especially if this is problematic substance use, many studies report that there are significantly lower levels of reunification in comparison to other groups where no substance use is present (Cheng, 2010, McGlade et al., 2009, Delfabbro et al., 2009, Murphy et al., 2017). Promisingly, studies have demonstrated that treatment for SUD in mothers increased reunification rates between 44% to 60% (Grella et al., 2009, Grant et al., 2011). However, a different study from Choi et al. (2012) demonstrated lower reunification rates of 26.9% overall. Higher reunification rates were found for mothers who were older (33.25% versus. 31.74%), who had ever married (37.0% versus 25.9%), and who had an education beyond high school completion (31.95% versus 23.9%).

The removal of a child into OOHC care is a very traumatic experience for mothers, families, and health and social care workers who work in this space (Hinton, 2018, Ross et al., 2017). While there is limited research on mothers' experiences of child removal, an emerging body of literature describes 'collateral consequences' for mothers when a child is removed from their care. (Broadhurst and Mason, 2019, Hinton, 2018, Broadhurst and Mason, 2013, Ross et al., 2017). Collateral consequences include feelings of despair, overwhelming grief and loss and reductions in income and housing instability. Additionally, women are expected to deal with legal processes, navigate complex welfare systems and meet any conditions imposed by child protection services and court orders (Hinton, 2018).

A literature review (Doab et al., 2015) undertaken as prior to commencement of this PhD thesis found that several factors contribute to higher reunification levels amongst mothers with a SUD.

These factors are timeliness of treatment entry, treatment completion, and receipt of matched services and programs that provide a greater level of integrated care. Conversely, barriers to reunification are the presence of a mental health disorder, opiate use and having a greater number of children. In addition, this review found that mothers with a SUD history and having a child in OOHC have multiple unmet needs such as concurrent mental health disorders. Recommendations to address these needs include improved access to stigma-free comprehensive, integrated care services and greater access to primary health care (PHC) that simultaneously addresses social and medical issues.

This literature review differs than the literature review within the main body of the thesis as it focusses solely on reunification of mothers who have experience child removal. As this research assisted me to refine my research question and focus for the PhD it is included as an appendix. See Appendix 1

Aboriginal women
It is well documented that health and social outcomes for Aboriginal mothers and babies are overall worse than their non-Aboriginal counterparts. These include increased maternal mortality (13.8 versus 6.6 deaths per 1,00,000 women), preterm birth (140 versus 80 per 1,000 births), low birth weight (118 versus 62 per 1,000 births) and perinatal deaths (14 versus 9 per 1,000 births) (AIHW, 2017b). Aboriginal women are also less likely to attend antenatal care in the first trimester compared to non-Aboriginal women (53% versus 60%) or to attend five or more antenatal visits overall (86% versus 95%) (AIHW, 2017b).

Some of the reasons for the discrepancies in health outcomes include a higher rate of teenage mothers (15% versus 2%), residing in remote/very remote areas (22% versus 1.6%), smoking during pregnancy (44% versus 12%) and higher rates of obesity and other pre-existing health conditions (AIHW, 2017b). Aboriginal women are also at risk of high rates of mental illness, increased substance use issues, and transgenerational trauma (NDARC 2015). Therefore, health professionals play a critical role in optimising the care of Aboriginal pregnant women to aid in 'closing the gap' in health outcomes. Practising cultural safety and providing culturally safe, holistic antenatal care is an essential factor in health care delivery and can improve outcomes for Aboriginal people (NDARC, 2015).

Infant-mother attachment

Attachment theory, an empirically grounded theory related to parenting, is based on the work by Bowlby and Ainsworth (Benoit, 2004). One of its principal tenants is that a child needs at least one primary caregiver that makes them feel safe and fosters social and emotional growth (Bretherton, 1992). Bowlby J (1969/1982) described attachment as the relationship between an infant and its caregiver that is the foundation for further healthy development. This attachment, mainly to the mother, provides a secure base for the baby to explore their world safely. Babies whose mothers and caregivers are sensitive and responsive to their needs are more likely to develop this secure base (Bowlby, 1988). A secure base leads to increased development of trust, resilience, and confidence as they mature (Ainsworth, 1979). Conversely, babies without a secure base can become anxious and mistrustful of their world, which can be problematic in later life (Ainsworth, 1979).

The presence of a SUD in a mother can negatively impact infant-mother attachment. Substance abuse can be associated with a dysregulation of reward and stress neurobiological systems. This dysregulation can lead to parenting with reduced sensitivity and lower responsiveness to infant cues, which are viewed as stressful instead (Parolin and Simonelli, 2016). These infants store memories or psychological 'representations' of these early caregiving experiences. These memories are thought to become the 'prototype' for newly formed relationships, including the next generation of caregiving relationships (Suchman et al., 2010). In addition, as children, they are at greater risk of developing behavioural problems such as disruptiveness that may continue into adolescence and adulthood (Godinet et al., 2014). As these children progress through life, they may be labelled as problematic children, and they are at higher risk of substance abuse themselves as adults (Solis et al., 2012).

Considering the effects of an insecure or dysfunctional infant-mother attachment can be life-long, urgent evidence-based strategies are required. Programs that offer attachment-based interventions for mothers with SUD are especially relevant. These programs directly promote sensitive, emotionally supportive parenting behaviours linked to child attachment security and address mothers' attachment traumas (Berlin et al., 2014). Evidence has found that these programs hold promise and may be more effective than traditional parent education for enhancing relationships between substance-using women and their young children (Berlin et al., 2014, Suchman et al., 2010). Furthermore, they may have particular leverage for breaking intergenerational cycles of maltreatment (Berlin et al., 2014).

Gender-specific treatment of substance use disorders

Substance use disorder treatment can mitigate some issues associated with parental substance use (Greenfield, Brooks et al. 2007). Since the 1970s there has been an interest in women's only substance use treatment settings, as women have different treatment needs than men (Ashley et al., 2003). In addition, as women are often the primary carers for their children, many women may find it challenging to find suitable treatment in the first place (Greenfield, Brooks et al. 2007).

While gender is not a significant predictor of treatment retention or completion, there is a consensus for greater access to gender-specific and pregnancy-specific treatment for women with SUDs (Hines, 2013). Gender-specific treatment can address issues specific to subpopulations of women, such as those who are pregnant or parenting (Greenfield et al., 2007, Niccols et al., 2012). For example, a systematic review by Ashley et al. (2003) examined the extent and effectiveness of substance abuse treatment programs for mothers and found that programs providing prenatal care and childcare have better outcomes for mothers and their children. This study includes data from women who were either pregnant, women with children or women with children regardless of parenting status. Another study noted that treatment that allows women to remain with their children whilst in residential care increased treatment retention and completion (Chen, Burgdorf et al. 2004). While treatment programs vary overall, programs of at least six months duration are associated with higher levels of abstinence (Conners et al., 2006, Greenfield et al., 2004).

Integrated women's only treatment can improve a women's sense of self, increase personal agency, and increase women's ability to recognise destructive behaviour patterns. Women also benefited from giving and receiving social support and self-disclosure of challenges, feelings and past experiences (Sword et al., 2009). In addition, having their children with them in treatment was a motivating factor and assisted women in their overall recovery (Sword et al., 2009). On a personal level, women with SUDs have stated that they prefer women's only services and they described feeling safer (Hines, 2013) and a sense of solace and belonging (Godlaski et al., 2009, Neale et al., 2018). At times though, tension between women would occur, especially if women felt others were gossiping about them (Godlaski et al., 2009, Neale et al., 2018).

Despite benefits of women's only SUD treatment, a review of women's only drug and alcohol services in NSW identified a lack of available and appropriate treatment services for women with children. This review undertaken in 2012 by the Network of Alcohol and Drugs Agency (NADA) (Jenner et al., 2014) found there were waiting lists for treatment entry and a lack of programs providing OAT. Programs provided inconsistent support for women with DCJ involvement and insufficient care for women with trauma and mental health histories. In addition, there was a requirement for care than met diverse population needs, such as Aboriginal women and culturally diverse women (Jenner et al., 2014).

Support for pregnant women with SUDs

Health care professionals can make a substantial difference to the outcomes of women with a SUD and their babies by identifying and supporting these women during pregnancy (NDARC, 2015). Well-coordinated and comprehensive support with early access to antenatal care and specialist treatment can reduce harm and improve outcomes for pregnant women with SUDs (SAMHSAb, 2021). Care teams must possess knowledge and skills to employ specific treatments and supports for women's substance use, including counselling, pharmacotherapies, and relapse prevention strategies (NSW Health, 2014). To develop rapport, it is important to avoid stigma and judgment and work within a culturally competent framework for Aboriginal women. Women identified as at risk of adverse outcomes due to SUDs must be referred for specialist antenatal care and consultation (NDARC, 2015, WHO, 2014).

Clinical practice care guidelines exist in Australia to guide practice for pregnant women with SUDs. These guidelines by NSW Health (NSW Health, 2014), the National Centre of Drug and Alcohol Research (NDARC) (NDARC, 2015), the Department of Health (DoH, 2016) and the Royal Australian and New Zealand College of General (RANZCOG) (RANZCOG, 2018), will be examined as part of this thesis, as there does not appear to be a review of these guidelines for practice.

The origins of this research

I am a clinical nurse consultant who has worked with pregnant women and mothers with SUDs for over 15 years. I work in an NSW Health lead PHC service in an inner-city Sydney suburb, Kings Cross. Historically, Kings Cross was known for its bohemian and arts culture and its connection to drugs, sex, and the underworld. It was a place you could buy 'sly grog' during the prohibition in the early part of the 19th Century and access sex workers that worked in bars and along the streets at the time. Moving forward to the 1960s, the 'Cross', as it is also known, was frequented by many American navy servicemen as they stayed at the navy port nearby. Consequently, sex work, drugs and alcohol continued to be a prominent feature alongside many sex shops and strip clubs that were highly visible along the main artery road, Darlinghurst Road.

In the 1980s, at a time when the HIV/AIDS crisis hit, there was a growing recognition that the needs of sex workers were not met, there were few acceptable health care options, and if nothing was done, there was a risk that the HIV/AIDS would further spread. In April 1987, in response to the NSW Select Committee of the Legislative Assembly Upon Prostitution (NSW, 1986), it was recommended that the NSW Government fund a multi-purpose health centre in the Kings Cross area. The Committee recognised that existing sexually transmitted disease (STD), now called sexually transmitted Infections (STIs), clinics and health care centres were not well adapted to the needs of sex workers, and it was proposed that these problems could be overcome by establishing a centre with a more flexible approach; with drop-in services and an outreach model that would be fully accessible and acceptable to sex workers. This centre would not be solely identified with an STD clinic and would also offer general health care, counselling, and other relevant services (NSW Government, 2015).

Kirketon Road Centre (KRC) was born. Kirketon Road Centre (KRC) is a walk-in, targeted PHC service operating since 1987. Kirketon Road Centre provides high quality, non-judgmental, free and confidential health care (Rodgers, 2012). The centre offers medical, counselling, and social welfare services to the target populations: young people, sex workers, PWID, people from lesbian, gay, bisexual, transgender and other gender diverse groups, Aboriginal people, and those experiencing homelessness. Typically, KRC provides services to around 4000 people per year.

During my time at KRC, and working with women who were injecting drugs, many of these women became pregnant over time, with many already having children living in OOHC. Women frequently did not engage in timely care, and they often went 'underground' whilst pregnant. They would resurface later on in their pregnancy, and there appeared to be a lot of trauma in their lives. Many continued to use drugs whilst pregnant and some engaged in sex work late into their pregnancy.

Babies were almost always removed straight from the hospital, and women would then spiral deeper into drug use, and many of their health and social needs appeared unmet. Some women would become pregnant again, and others would not be seen for a long time, or not again. Given the crisis nature of much of the work undertaken at KRC, staff would hope that if a woman was not seen in or around KRC or Kings Cross, it was because they were relatively stable. However, ultimately some women would return, sometimes in crisis, sometimes pregnant again, and continue the cycle.

My research question was developed as a direct result of my work and observations at KRC: What are the needs and experiences of pregnant women and new mothers with a history of IDU?

Additionally, I discussed this topic with Associate Professor Carolyn Day from the University of Sydney, Addiction Medicine, Central Clinical School, who supported me and encouraged me to explore this question as a PhD thesis.

Outline of thesis

Chapter one provides an overview of the current situation of substance use and IDU both from an International and an Australian perspective. This chapter describes the definitions and patterns of substance abuse and policy responses and treatments of SUD. Health and social outcomes of PWID are discussed, including sections on mothers and substance use, child protection and out of home care outcomes. There is a section on Aboriginal mothers as a priority group. Finally, gender-specific treatment for substance use disorders is examined.

Chapter two is a qualitative meta-synthesis literature review. It aimed to provide an in-depth understanding of the health care experiences of pregnant and parenting women with SUDs, the sociocultural factors that influence access to SUD treatment, as well as the needs of pregnant women who had children in their care and were in SUD treatment.

Chapter three describes the rationale for the study, the aims of the study and the research questions.

Chapter four provides a description of the theoretical framework, methodology and procedures that were employed to conduct this study. Details of the study design and setting, study population, recruitment and consent procedures, data collection and analysis and the study's ethical considerations are presented.

Chapter five presents findings from the background study, which consists of the service review and the guideline review. The service review describes the types of residential services available to support pregnant women and new mothers with SUDs and the clinical guidelines to support their care when engaging in health care services.

Chapters six and seven presents the results from the quantitative interviews that were conducted with the women. This includes demographics, health status, substance use history, the number of children, and their child protection history. Results from standardised measures that were taken are included in this chapter. The findings from the qualitative interviews that were conducted with the women are discussed in chapter seven.

Chapters eight and nine both describe the findings from the qualitative interviews that were conducted with the health and social care providers and the Department of Community Service workers.

Chapter ten discusses the study findings and examines how they relate to the aims of the study and research questions, the background literature and qualitative review. This chapter also addresses the study's limitations and concludes with a consideration of the implications of the study for research and practice and recommendations.

CHAPTER TWO: LITERATURE REVIEW

Introduction

Quality health care interactions and satisfactory experiences lead to treatment uptake and improved health outcomes (Levesque et al., 2013). Women may engage with health services for many reasons. For pregnant women with SUDs, pregnancy can be a strong motivator to reduce their drug use, enter and stay in treatment, and engage in pregnancy care (Olszewski, 2009, Olsen et al., 2012). Pregnancy provides an opportunity for professionals to foster a positive rather than a punitive approach to caring for this population of women at risk of IPV, mental health issues, poverty and homelessness (Metz et al., 2012). Women may also be motivated to engage in care to mitigate feelings of guilt associated with the possibility that their baby may experience NAS, for example (Mahoney et al., 2019). However, women may have a negative experience with these services, which may dissuade them from seeking continuing care.

Women-focused SUD treatment can benefit women (Ashley et al., 2003). It can increase retention and treatment completion for pregnant or parenting women (Greenfield, Brooks et al. 2007) by allowing these women to remain with their children whilst in residential care (Chen et al., 2004). It is important to view consumer perception of access to health care, especially for marginalised and vulnerable populations, as these groups can find it difficult to articulate their health care needs due to unique challenges such as low health literacy (Richard et al., 2016). These unique challenges can lead to a lack of understanding of the specific needs of women, resulting in a paucity of appropriate drug treatment services that take into account the diverse needs of women with SUDs (UNODC, 2018). Multiple barriers to treatment exist for pregnant, and parenting women and many services do not accommodate children (Jessup et al., 2003).

A literature review from 2003 of programs to support women with SUDs who were pregnant or parenting found that programs that provide prenatal care and childcare have better outcomes for mothers and children (Ashley et al., 2003). A different review of 30 studies from 1992-2010, which described the substance abuse treatment views and recommendations of substance-using mothers, found that pregnant and parenting women preferred gender-specific services. Women described feeling safer in women only services and they felt more comfortable discussing issues such as sexual abuse, the removal of one's children into care or their sex work (Hines 2013).

As these reviews were undertaken several years ago, there is a need to explore a more contemporary view of health care experiences of both pregnant and parenting women who are attempting to engage, or are engaged with SUD treatment programs, so we can understand their needs, values and preferences for care. In addition, it is necessary to understand their experiences and interactions, so a comprehensive overview of the context of care can be provided. This knowledge is essential to planning new services and evaluating current ones to improve the quality of care and services for this vulnerable population.

A meta-synthesis of the qualitative literature was undertaken to gain an up-to-date and in-depth understanding of the treatment and health care experiences of pregnant and parenting women with SUDs.

Methods

A qualitative meta-synthesis design was used to explore the experiences of pregnant women and mothers with SUDs engaging in health care or engaging in a SUD treatment program. Meta-syntheses are useful to examine phenomena such as experiences and to understand the effects of the environment, the organisation, individual factors, the effects of a clinical intervention and the complex interactions that these have on one another (Dawson, 2019). The analyses of the findings of qualitative studies allows space for new insights and understandings to emerge that can inform policy and improve patient care (Finfgeld, 2003) The Levesque et al. (2013) framework of health access and interactions was used to examine the literature and to provide structure to the review (Grant and Osanloo, 2014).

The review question was developed using the PICO framework (Population, Intervention, Comparison, Outcome) (Schardt et al., 2007): '(P) For women with a substance use disorder who are either pregnant or parenting and trying to engage or are engaged (I) in health care and, or SUD treatment programs, (O) how do they experience the treatment and services provided to them?'. The comparison component was not applied in this situation and is not always necessary or applicable (Huang et al., 2006).

Search strategy
The following databases were searched: PubMed, Embase, CINAHL, Psychinfo, Medline, Scopus, Web of Science, Google Scholar, and hand searching of reference lists within relevant published literature. The following key search terms and their synonyms were used singularly and in

combination and with both USA and UK/AUS spelling where applicable: 'substance-related disorders', 'pregnancy', 'mothers', 'rehabilitation', 'women', 'health care', 'perinatal', 'children', 'substance abuse treatment', 'opioid use treatment', 'opioid use disorder', 'residential treatment', 'experiences'. As there is a need for a contemporary review, only articles between 2008-2020 were selected to be examined for review, and they must have met the following inclusion criteria: 1) qualitative studies (or mixed methods with a large qualitative component); 2) studies that examined experiences of pregnant women engaging in perinatal care; and/or 3) studies that examined experiences of women either accessing or engaged in SUD treatment. This SUD treatment could be in an inpatient setting such as rehabilitation or a community outpatient treatment setting such as an OAT setting; 4) Women must be pregnant or parenting. The definition of experiences was broad and included barriers, facilitators, needs or similar. If papers provided data sources such as health care workers, only the women's perspectives were included. The PRISMA diagram demonstrated the search process (Moher et al., 2009). See Diagram 1.

Quality Appraisal

Papers were appraised using the Critical Appraisal Skills Programme (CASP) Qualitative review checklist (CASP 2018). This checklist was used to assess the quality of the articles for inclusion. The checklists contain ten questions (items) that guide researchers to review qualitative studies to assess their validity and utility (see Appendix 2). All appraised studies were of sufficient quality to be included in the analysis.

Diagram 1: Prisma diagram

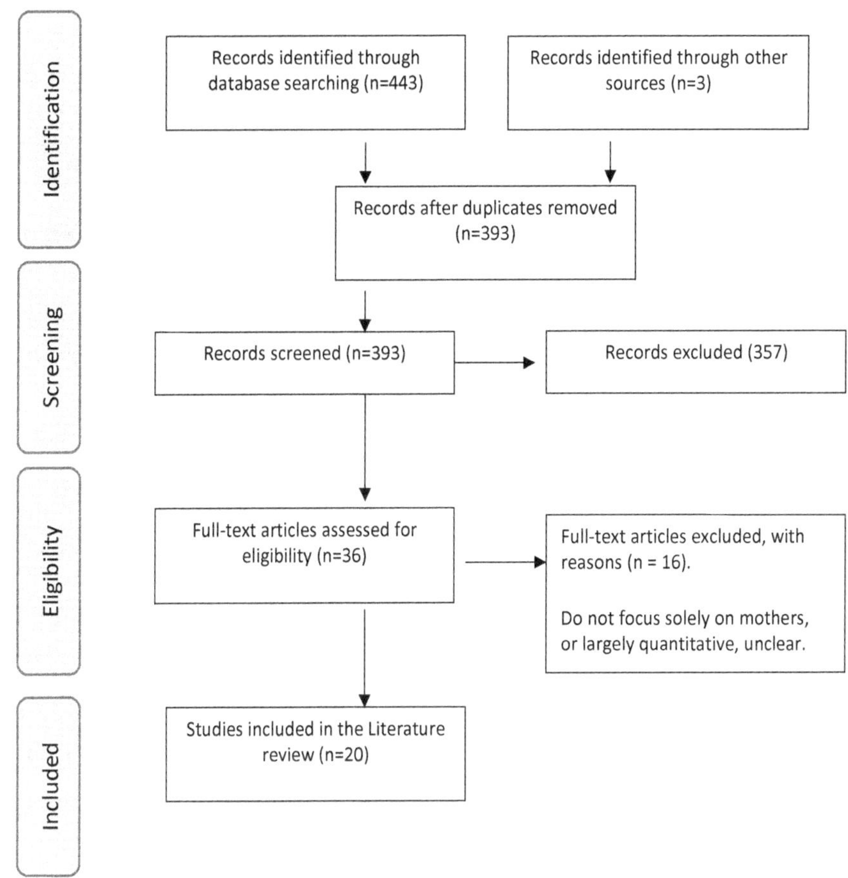

Data extraction and analysis

A textual narrative analysis was undertaken by extracting data (quotations) from each paper's results and discussion sections (Pope et al., 2000). These data were read line by line and examined for relevancy to the research question. Only data pertinent to the women's experiences and/or described health care interactions were included for analysis (Thomas and Harden, 2008). These extractions were tabulated where patterns were identified, and themes grouped. Emerging patterns and textual themes were further explored through the manual creation of a concept map. This assisted in exploring patterns, themes and relationships across studies. An inductive approach to the analysis was conducted where the data forms the findings from the ground up (Nowell et al., 2017).

The Levesque framework for health care access was applied to interpret the findings to provide structure, offer new insights into health care experiences, and suggestions for improvement (Levesque et al., 2013). This framework goes beyond the traditional view of access which is often defined as the opportunity in which consumers can use appropriate services in proportion to their needs, but also includes a person's ability to interact with a health care service (Levesque et al., 2013).

According to Levesque et al. (2013) there are five paired dimensions of health care access which are: 1) Approachability and ability to perceive; 2) Acceptability and ability to seek; 3) Availability and accommodation and ability to reach; 4) Affordability and ability to pay, and 5) Appropriateness and ability to engage. These paired dimensions operate as a supply-demand dichotomy. Supply includes the location, availability, or cost of services, and demand consists of the burden of disease and knowledge, attitudes and skills and self-care practices of the population (Levesque et al., 2013). These dimensions are not discrete and can influence each other and can occur at various times during an episode of care (Levesque et al., 2013). This framework is relevant to marginalised and vulnerable populations and those with chronic diseases such as SUDs (Richard et al., 2016).

Findings

Overview of studies

Twenty papers were included in the review (See Appendix 3). Fourteen studies were from the USA; two were from Sydney, Australia one each from Canada, Scotland, Israel and New Zealand. Across the included studies, 413 women were either pregnant or parenting at the time of interview. Two studies described in this review (Jackson and Shannon 2012, Jackson and Shannon 2013) are from the same cohort of 114 women and therefore are counted once in the overall tally of women.

The included studies provided insight into women's experiences of perinatal care, inpatient drug treatment programs, outpatient treatment and mixed treatment settings, and access to SUD treatment. Three studies focused on perinatal care experiences for women with SUDs within hospital settings. Of these, one explored 32 women's perceptions of prenatal drug and alcohol screening (Roberts and Nuru-Jeter, 2010), and two studies examined the experiences of Mexican-American mothers of infants with NAS in the neonatal intensive care unit (Cleveland and Gill, 2013, Cleveland and Bonugli, 2014). The study from 2014 was a secondary analysis of the same cohort of women, where five out of the initial 15 women described a more difficult overview of the issues which needed further exploration.

Two studies focused on the barriers, facilitators and motivations women experienced when accessing SUD treatment. Gueta (2017) explored the experiences of care access for 25 substance-using Israeli mothers and Jackson and Shannon (2012) examined experiences of 114 rural and urban pregnant women entering a short-term detoxification program.

Women's experiences of inpatient drug treatment programs were examined in four studies. Eindbinder (2009), examined 21 mothers' experiences of family-friendly long term residential settings, Thompson et al. (2013) examined the experiences of 27 mothers who were participating in the Partners in Recovery program, which is a court-mandated program. Jackson and Shannon (2013) examined perceptions of substance abuse treatments and motivation for entering treatment, while Wong (2008) focused on the parenting experience of mothers with children in residential drug treatment programs.

Eight studies focused on pregnant and parenting women's experiences in outpatient treatment settings. Of these, two studies examined the experiences of support groups for women on OAT. Chandler et al. (2013) interviewed 12 mothers and Mattocks et al. (2017) interviewed 14 women; five women were pregnant, and nine were post-partum. In addition, one study examined experiences of outpatient care for 17 women with depression with SUD and who were on OAT (Kuo et al., 2013), and another study by (Lefebvre et al., 2010) examined experiences of prenatal care of 19 women at an integrated care outpatient setting.

Finney Lamb et al. (2008) examined experiences of 13 mothers on OAT and the provision of child and midwifery services, and their ability to make health care provider complaints. Chan (2010) explored the experiences of five pregnant women in an outpatient OAT program, and Harvey et al. (2015) examined perceptions of health care of six mothers who were on an OAT program who had newborn babies. Demirci et al. (2015) examined perceptions surrounding breastfeeding decisions among seven pregnant women and four post-partum women on methadone.

The final three studies explored experiences of pregnant women and new mothers in various settings. Linton et al. (2009) explored the experiences of 23 women participating in an aftercare program of a drug treatment program. These women had participated in a mix of inpatient and outpatient treatment detoxification programs. Another study recruited post-partum women (up to six months) from hospitals and drug treatment settings. The study's goal was to examine how women with an opioid use disorder and are pregnant participate in medical decision making, particularly concerning their prenatal and post-partum care, their opiate use and their perceptions of their own decision making (Howard, 2016). Finally, Stone (2015) conducted interviews with 30 recently pregnant women who had used alcohol or other drugs during their pregnancies. These women had participated in different treatment settings, including residential settings, prisons, OAT and detoxification centres (Stone, 2015).

Sociodemographic characteristics of women

The mothers' ages were not reported in the following studies (Chan, 2010, Cleveland and Gill, 2013, Kuo et al., 2013, Linton et al., 2009, Thompson et al., 2013) but where ages were reported in the other studies, women ranged from 19-48 years. All women were either pregnant or parenting, and the ages of children ranged from newborn to 16 years of age. Where reported, women were largely from metropolitan areas, except in the studies by Jackson and Shannon, (2012) and (2013), where, of the 114 women, 75% were from a rural area. In one study, Kuo et al. (2013) reported outcomes of 17 women who all scored high on the Edinburgh Postnatal Depression Scale, meaning that they were at risk of or had levels of depression that were distressing. Not all studies reported ethnicity, but overall, the main identities were Caucasian, African American, and Hispanic. Ethnic or cultural identity was not reported in the Australian or New Zealand studies. In the Israeli study, the women were mostly second-generation immigrant Mizrahi families.

Themes

Seven themes emerged as central to the women's health care experiences engaging in SUD treatment. These were: 1) Stigma and judgment, 2) Fear and guilt and subtheme of power and control, 3) Treatment burden and misconceptions, 4) We're poor, 5) Bringing children with me, 6) Learning how to be mum, and 7) Empowerment.

Stigma and judgment

Mothers across 11 studies described the stigma they felt as pregnant women or mothers with a SUD. Stigma was experienced when accessing treatment (Jackson and Shannon, 2012, Gueta, 2017), when their babies were in the neonatal intensive care ward (Cleveland and Gill, 2013, Cleveland and Bonugli, 2014), whilst receiving OAT (Stone, 2015, Mattocks et al., 2017, Chandler et al., 2013, Finney Lamb et al., 2008, Harvey et al., 2015, Chan, 2010) and while engaging in mainstream health care services such as in a hospital or emergency care unit (Lefebvre et al., 2010).

In the study by (Chan, 2010), women felt that health care workers judged them because of their history of substance use. One woman said that she felt that care providers focused only on her as a drug user and nothing else. She quoted, 'My doctor, he didn't want to know me. He just…put me to the high risk people' (Chan, 2010 p.66). Members of the public also judged women. One study described that a women was spoken to negatively by a member of the public, which is evidenced by the following remark; 'You get folk looking at you … whether I've got [my older child] with me or not, so it's just, there's the junkie, look at her' (Chandler et al., 2013 p.40).

Cleveland and Bonugli (2014) interviewed 15 mothers of children with NAS, and they all felt stigmatised during their time in hospital. One woman described how one nurse said the following about her newborn who was in withdrawal; 'You're going to have a lot of problems with that little baby because he's real jumpy and jittery, his muscles are locking up because of his junkie mom' Cleveland and Bonugli (2014 p.324). In this study, women spoke about their life stories and what had led them to addiction. One woman said that she felt that if the nurses were more educated and had a greater understanding of mothers' histories, this may help.

Another woman described her experiences as feeling like no one knew the real her, which echoes the sentiment of the women in the study by Chan (2010). She felt like turning around and saying the following to the nurse; 'Do you know me? Do you really know me? (Cleveland and Bonugli, 2014 p.324). As a consequence of these judgements, women were worried that this led to their babies scoring higher on the NAS score and that the score was contingent on whether the nurse liked them. If the nurse liked them, they would get a 'better' score than if they did not (Cleveland and Gill, 2013).

Conversely, some interactions with care providers were positive, as one woman described her social worker's profound effect on her. 'After giving birth, I hadn't seen my son for four days… I didn't know what he looked like … she [the social worker] put me in a wheelchair and took me to the nursery to see my baby' (Gueta, 2017 p.160). In the study by (Lefebvre et al., 2010) which examines perceptions of an integrated model of care for substance abuse in pregnancy, they found that a non-judgmental atmosphere that enabled them to feel comfortable disclosing their substance use was important. One woman stated, 'I liked her a lot because she wasn't judging '(Lefebvre et al., 2010 p.50).

Fear and guilt

Women described being fearful of authorities and what may happen if they were exposed to be using drugs. At times this meant they did not divulge to health care providers about their substance use, and for some, they would make efforts to avoid interactions with health care providers (Roberts and Nuru-Jeter, 2010, Stone, 2015). In the study by (Stone, 2015), where they examined experiences of mothers with SUDs as they navigated health and criminal justice systems, one woman commented 'that stuff [the drugs] lasts in your system for three to four days, so I would make sure not to do it [use drugs] around the time of the appointment, just to be on the safe side' (Stone, 2015 p.8).

Roberts and Nuru-Jeter (2010) reported similar experiences of women fearing being 'found out', and again, they did not attend antenatal appointments if they had recently used drugs. The non-attendance of appointments or rearranging appointments also stemmed from the fact that women felt ashamed and guilty about using substances while pregnant. Women felt that it was hard for anyone who had not used drugs (such as the doctors) to be able to understand their situations (Roberts and Nuru-Jeter, 2010). Phrases such as 'guilt,' 'shame,' 'embarrassment', and 'undeserving' were used to describe feelings related to being identified as a substance user (Roberts and Nuru-Jeter, 2010).

Women expressed guilt and confusion about the benefits of OAT in pregnancy. One woman felt that she was being punished for her drug use and having to stay on methadone was the punishment. She said: 'I had already been on methadone for four months when I found out I was pregnant, and I was like; "Oh I have to get off methadone". And then I felt like they were punishing me'… (Mattocks et al., 2017 p.648). This confusion was illustrated in a different study that examined barriers and motivators to enter treatment. One woman said I thought to myself 'I want off this methadone…cause I didn't want to be on methadone while pregnant again' (Jackson and Shannon, 2012 p.575).

Women also feared child protection officers and were worried that their children could be removed into OOHC. This fear, at times, influenced their treatment decisions and compelled women to access SUD treatment. This is evidence by the following comment, 'The judge told me I was going to lose my daughter if I didn't do something' (Jackson and Shannon, 2012 p.575). When this women was asked what she hoped the treatment would help her achieve in the long-term?, she replied; 'not risk losing her son' (Jackson and Shannon, 2012 p.575). Another woman who had participated in the Partners in Recovery Program, a court-mandated program, agreed to do so as it was 'the only way to keep my kids' (Thompson et al., 2013 p.146). In this study, some women had said that attending substance use treatment had little to do with a desire to obtain sobriety but because they would do whatever it took to try to be reunited or remain with their children. In a different study that examines motivations for treatment, one mother who was a single mother who had lost custody of three of her four children also described the fear of the repercussions if she did not enter treatment. She said; 'I was dead inside, I knew I needed a solution, treatment…I thought if they took the baby, I would really die this time' (Gueta, 2017 p.158).

For women who had a history of a child removed into care after disclosing substance use, trust was even more difficult to establish. Again, women felt sometimes they remained silent about their level of substance use for fear that their child would be removed (Roberts and Nuru-Jeter, 2010). Mitigating factors were when women were praised for decreasing use, which made it easier for them to engage in care and eased their guilt (Roberts and Nuru-Jeter, 2010).

Sub-theme: Power and Control
Stemming from fear, women were subdued and felt powerless to ask questions or speak out when they did not understand their situations. Women describe feeling undermined or worried about speaking out for fear of the repercussions of doing so. One woman said the following about her meeting with her social worker 'Either you go the TC (Therapeutic community), or you won't see your son anymore. And then she said goodbye. She didn't explain anything about the community and I didn't know what it was' (Gueta, 2017 p.159). In this study, another mother described how a negative interaction with a service provider made her more determined to succeed. She stated that she had to undertake a parental competence test, which was 'negative'. It annoyed me so much, I said: 'definitely not; I'm going to try and that's it' (Gueta, 2017 p.159).

A different woman described feeling undermined by a controlling nurse, and she felt that this had an impact on her mothering abilities. This demonstrates the power that health care providers have over these women at times. This woman said, 'She wouldn't let me change her diaper. She wouldn't let me hold her. She wouldn't let me do anything. And whenever I finally said I want to breastfeed her, [the nurse] just to show me, she just said; 'Okay, take [your breast] out' and she just put the baby's head there and that was it. She walked out of the room' (Demirci et al., 2015 p.206).

The lack of power that women felt when encountering health care interactions was noted in another study that described the experiences and attitudes of opioid-dependent women regarding making health care complaints during pregnancy and early motherhood. Of the 11 out of 14 women interviewed, they remained silent, even when they were unhappy with health care experiences within the child and maternity services. One mother was quoted as saying; 'You're just so scared that they're going to take your baby off you. You just do what they tell you to. It's like they're playing God…'(Finney Lamb et al., 2008 p.69).

Treatment burden and misconceptions
At times, women found treatment burdensome. For example, getting to the treatment centre and then waiting for the methadone to take effect took time. One woman reported, 'It takes about an hour, maybe an hour and a half for my meth [methadone] to kick in … I don't remember what it's

like to wake up [normal]' (Chandler et al., 2013 p.40). Other misconceptions about the role of methadone were described in the study by Stone (2015) where several women described it as 'liquid handcuffs' (Stone, 2015 p.10). Despite this, it was acknowledged by one woman as a necessary treatment to move forward; 'now I look at it differently, I'm glad it was there to change my life' (Stone, 2015 p.10).

Other treatment types, such as therapy sessions, were criticised by some women as being difficult to adhere to, and they felt the expectations were too high. One woman noted that there were 'too many therapy sessions… to add an hour of like individual counselling to my schedule is not gonna happen' (Kuo et al., 2013 p.1502). Another participant described this challenge in the following way: 'I'm already doing it [therapy] at three different places…' (Kuo et al., 2013 p.1502).

Misconceptions were noted about methadone and breastfeeding. One woman was concerned that her baby may 'overdose', become 'high', or go into withdrawal' (Demirci et al., 2015 p.4). Some women also feared that their baby would become hepatitis C positive through breastfeeding. One woman noted that she had never seen this happen, but she had heard about this happening and so could not get the thought out of her head (Demirci et al., 2015).

Some women who had a baby with NAS described the guilt and anguish of observing their baby going through withdrawals, and felt like they were 'bad mothers' (Harvey et al., 2015). A mother whose daughter was given phenobarbitone, a barbiturate sometimes used to treat NAS, stated, 'Watching my daughter go through it? Yeah, that's bad. It really woke me up, I want to come off methadone…It wasn't fair to her' (Stone, 2015 p.11). Guilt was also mentioned in the context of sobriety. Being free of substances provided clarity over their situation as they realised the impacts that their drug use had on their children (Wong, 2008).

Relationships with child protective services were strained for some women, as they felt that they could never do anything right, even when they felt they were doing well. This is evidenced by the following quote: 'They need to focus more on what we are doing right instead of what we're doing wrong… She never focuses on what I have accomplished' (Thompson et al., 2013 p.149). Being on a SUD treatment program also meant that some women felt they were under surveillance, and being on a program left them more vulnerable to being reported (Howard, 2016).

We're poor
Some women were impacted by poverty, making it difficult to access and remain in SUD treatment. One woman from Israel, who, due to her immigrant status meant she had no health insurance,

noted the following: 'I wanted to go to rehab so someone would take care of us, but you need
health insurance and money, which we didn't have' (Gueta, 2017 p.159). Another Israeli immigrant
also found it challenging to enter treatment without health insurance. She was offered access to
treatment by a stranger. She said: '[He] told me there was a rehab project. [He said] "I will arrange
rehab for you without money"...I had no money'. She was extremely grateful for this opportunity,
and she now had some 'hope' (Gueta, 2017 p.159).

Four studies from the USA also found that finances could impact treatment access and the ability to
remain in treatment. In the study by Jackson and Shannon (2012), which examined barriers and
motivators for treatments, they found that financial barriers to entering treatment were an issue for
some women who indicated that 'money' and 'good insurance' were issues, as were 'financial
worries' about paying for treatment. A different study from the USA that examined treatment
outcomes also found that women had financial concerns, which impacted their ability to access
treatment, physically get to treatment centres, and pay for treatment. This is demonstrated by the
following statement, 'Here's the thing. We're poor. We don't have cars. We don't have licenses...
We need the transportation' (Kuo et al., 2013 p.1503).

Some women who could access treatment felt nervous that their financial situation may change; for
example, their Medicaid may be cut off, and there would be no ongoing means to pay. One woman
was concerned that she may have to detox rapidly, which would harm her foetus if this was the case.
She noted, 'if they're not going to pay for it, I'm gonna have to get off of it a lot faster than would be
healthy [for the baby]' (Stone, 2015 p.11).

The impact of poverty on these women's lives was evident in more ways than accessing and
remaining in SUD treatment; it also included limited access to reproductive health services and
essential items such as food and clothing. One woman described the following: 'I wanted very much
to get rid of [the pregnancy]. When I found out I was pregnant, my world was destroyed, but I did
not have time to get an abortion... I also needed money.... To pay the abortion committee' (Gueta,
2017 p.159). In the study by Eindbinder (2009), the 21 women who completed an 18-month
residential rehabilitation centre expressed gratitude for being assisted with basic needs such as food
and clothing and being permitted to remain in treatment even when they had run out of money.
This demonstrates these women's difficulties meeting basic needs and the financial ability to remain
in treatment.

Bringing children with me

The role of children in treatment elicited mixed responses. Some women experienced barriers when attempting to enter a treatment program with their children, and some women found having their children with them helpful. In contrast, others found difficulties with having children in treatment. At times, women did not enter residential treatment services as they could not attend with their children. For example, one woman from Israel decided not to join a particular treatment service as she could not take her child; 'for me, it was because my older son could not come with me to the community' (Gueta, 2017 p.159). This difficulty in treatment access was echoed in a study by Eindbinder (2009) where a mother found herself in a similar scenario; 'We tried a few times [to access treatment] but could not bring our children with us' (Eindbinder, 2009 p.36).

Accessing SUD treatment with children was an important consideration for women attending outpatient programs. In the study by Kuo et al. (2013), 18 women with depression and a SUD were interviewed, women were grateful they could take their children to the treatment program. One woman noted the following 'What really helps is like if you have your kid, you can bring him here (Kuo et al., 2013 p.1503)

Some women in residential treatment, found having children with them difficult. Women commented on how badly their own children behaved and realised that this may have been because they had time to focus on them and notice their behaviour (Eindbinder, 2009), this made it difficult for these women to concentrate. This was a similar experience for women in the study by Linton et al. (2009). One mother commented, 'When you are busy focusing on the kids and their acting out it's hard to focus on yourself. Even more worrying, it was noted in one study that a child ended up being abused by other children who then had to leave the program to stay with other family members. This mother stated that the children were 'almost feral' (Stone, 2015 p.13).

Learning how to be mum

Women across several studies described how being in treatment led them to develop new skills such as being a better mother, staying 'clean', and insights into their own history and how this impacted their parenting. One woman commented that she could 'learn so much about yourself' (Linton et al., 2009 p.291). A different woman in court-mandated treatment learnt how 'to be clean?' (Kuo et al., 2013 p.1503). Being in the treatment itself was a motivating factor for women, and some women hoped that treatment would provide them with the knowledge to be 'a better mother' (Jackson and Shannon, 2013).

Mothers described being grateful for the parenting guidance they received as part of their treatment sessions. One woman stated 'I didn't really have any parenting skills so coming here with the help of parenting classes and everything, showed me things I was doing wrong and … how to do things in a different way' (Eindbinder, 2009 p.39). Another woman in the study by Wong (2008) spoke about treatment positively and how she developed a new appreciation for her child and their needs. One mother stated: '[I know] when they want more love, or for you to just hold them…and I wouldn't be conscious to respond to their needs if I were high' (Wong, 2008 p.171). Some mothers discussed that their personal histories of trauma and addiction had impacted their children; 'I know I wasn't always a great mom, and I didn't really know a lot of things about being a mother because I was never mothered myself' (Eindbinder, 2009 p.39). A different mother stated, 'I know if I didn't have an addiction, I probably would have been [a] better parent' (Eindbinder, 2009 p.39).

Once women were engaged in treatment, they became conscious of its benefits, and that they were able to think more clearly. Wong (2009) found that for women who attended a residential group, over time, felt connected to their children, especially after the effects of the drugs started to wear off. One woman spoke about how she felt she handled her son's behaviour better than she did with her elder child (Wong, 2008).

Being able to breastfeed was important for some women and alleviated some of the guilt associated with initial pregnancy ambivalence (Stone, 2015). The benefits of breastfeeding were also acknowledged; 'You know, even with my oldest son, I never really gave [breastfeeding] a chance. I let him try it one time, and I didn't like it, so it never happened again. But I'm trying to do what's best for my baby, because if my breast milk will help her from her withdrawals, then that's what I'm going to do.' (Stone, 2015 p.9). In this study, part of learning how to be mum was truth telling regarding their substance use and this honesty would demonstrate to the authorities they could be 'good' mothers who wanted to do the right thing for their children (Stone, 2015). Similarly, a different study found that some women who had used drugs throughout pregnancy still attended all appointments, even though they feared CPS reports. A primary motivator was their baby's health (Roberts and Nuru-Jeter, 2010), demonstrating commitment to their newborn infants and children, even if there was a risk of being identified as using drugs.

Empowerment
Despite the hardships that many women in these studies have faced, hope for the future was a prominent feature. Many women spoke about the 'lifestyle of recovery' and how this created hope and the opportunity to 'make a new start' (Thompson et al., 2013 p.149). One woman felt that the

program provided her with an opportunity to get back to her old self. 'I am excited about getting away from it. I really want to get my life back... (Jackson and Shannon, 2013 p. 337). Linton et al. (2009) described women as feeling empowered by the program that they were involved with and that the program involved 'learning about who I am, and that they were able to show their 'true self. One woman noted that 'the program focused on empowering rather than powerlessness; this makes it great!' (Linton et al., 2009 p.290). The program that these women were involved with was a 16-step (Kasl, 1994) holistic service that focused on empowerment.

Given that there were, at times, negative interactions with health care providers, some women were still in a position where they felt able to assert themselves and their role as a mother. Cleveland and Gill (2013) found that all five women, all of whom were Hispanic, identified that they were and should be the primary carers and decision-makers about their baby in the NICU. They felt frustrated and were resentful towards the staff when they felt that their needs were not being listened to. One woman said, 'I'm the mother here. I know what I'm doing' (Cleveland and Gill, 2013 p.323).

Women enjoyed the holistic nature of services (Eindbinder, 2009), and others spoke about the positive role that dedicated doctors had regarding their OAT. One woman described that she felt judged by mainstream hospital services but more comfortable in integrated care services for pregnant women and new mothers with SUDs. 'When I see my doctor here, it's different... I can see it in how my doctor looks at me. Somewhere else they don't look at you at all... here, they understand you . . . you're somebody' (Lefebvre et al., 2010 p.50). Not being judged was an important factor noted by women who valued being depicted as a person that can make positive change. Women felt more valued as a person when they felt they were respected and interactions were not laden with judgment and stigma. Cleveland and Bonugli (2014) noted the following: 'They understood [health care workers]. They didn't make me feel like an outcast. They made me feel very comfortable' (Cleveland and Bonugli, 2014 p.325).

Some suggestions for improvement offered by women included peer support in treatment, as women felt that it was difficult to relate to staff who did not have a history of a SUD (Thompson et al., 2013). A different study similarity noted that it was difficult to relate to staff. One woman said, 'I think one of the biggest challenges I'm having is having somebody who's not an addict try to teach you things' (Kuo et al., 2013 p.1502). A woman in another study again suggested that peer support may overcome this barrier. This woman noted that she would be '...more comfortable [with peer support] because you're around people who are sharing the same experience ... you're at ease to express your issues because people are going through the exact same thing as you' (Lefebvre et al.,

2010 p.51). In the study by Lefebvre et al. (2010), the women felt more valued and cared for when staff were supportive of their needs and were encouraging when they did well. This also meant that they felt more at ease and were more likely to engage in follow up care. This was more relevant to being the recipient of care by health professionals who specialise in working with mothers with SUDs. One woman expressed the difference in her care when she was accessing mainstream health care services instead of specialist care.

Discussion

Positive health care interactions and experiences are important factors for quality health care (Levesque et al., 2013). It was apparent in this review that health care experiences for women with SUDs who are pregnant, or parenting are mixed and are hindered by judgment, stigma, fear and misconceptions. This includes being judged and stigmatised by health care workers and fearing child protection authorities. In addition, women felt judged as incompetent mothers and described power imbalances between them and health service providers.

For some women, treatment was burdensome, and they felt guilty and ashamed of the effects that their substance use may have had on their newborns and children. Women, at times, had little trust in the system, and some women appeared to lack understanding of the role of treatment. Lack of trust may be due to a lack of health literacy, and treatment misconceptions. Some women experienced difficulties accessing treatment that met their individual needs. On the contrary, some women praised services for the new skills and knowledge they had acquired and were grateful when treated with respect and dignity (Linton et al., 2009, Eindbinder, 2009).

The Levesque framework (Levesque et al., 2013) guided the discussion. This assisted to describe women's experiences of health care access and offers insights into how care provision and outcomes can be improved.

Approachability and ability to perceive health care

This paired dimension of approachability and the ability to perceive health care relates to the ability of a woman to identify that a health service exists, it can be reached, and that it can have a positive impact on health (Levesque et al., 2013). This qualitative synthesis found that many women did not fully engage in health care for fear of being found out that they were 'drug users'; and that their children may be removed into care. This lack of engagement highlights the importance of positive relationships between clinicians and women when care-seeking and accessing appropriate services.

The women in the included studies also demonstrated low levels of knowledge about the benefits of methadone in pregnancy, which can potentially affect treatment uptake. These findings indicate the need to improve women's health literacy to enhance their ability to understand the benefits of treatment and seek care. Suggestions to improve health literacy in people with SUDs include the provision of psychoeducation using self-management strategies and emphasising skill-building (Degan et al., 2019). On the service side, it is recommended that staff be provided with education to understand the complexities of working with women with SUDs (Degan et al., 2019). In addition, health services could be better promoted, which may improve access by providing clear information about available treatments and services and outreach activities.

Acceptability and ability to seek care

This paired dimension relates to the influence that cultural and social factors play in determining the possibility for people to accept aspects of a service. This relates to personal autonomy, knowledge about health care options, and individual rights. Perceptions of stigma and discrimination play an important role here (Levesque et al., 2013). This review highlighted the services did not always meet the individual's needs. Women wanted more autonomy and choice in treatment options, and this included being able to take their children with them into treatment. Women also described feeling overburdened by the intensity of treatment sessions and did not always feel they were useful (Levesque et al., 2013).

Stigma and discrimination were *everyday* experiences by many women in this review, and they feared interactions with child protection workers and the risk of having their babies removed. Stigma has profound effects on the way that people with SUDs interact with health care as this group is often marginalised and stigmatised by society as a whole, but also health care workers (Brener et al., 2007b, Meyers et al., 2021, Nyblade et al., 2019). Adverse outcomes of this stigma include lower rates of treatment access and completion (Brener et al., 2010), which impacts an individual's mental and physical health (Ahern et al., 2007). Women with SUDs and mothers are doubly stigmatised as it goes against the ideals of femininity and being a nurturer and carer (Lee and Boeri, 2017).

Consequences of stigma and fear for women in this review meant that women would sometimes present late to care or avoid or disengage from care altogether. This is a commonly cited issue for women with SUDs engaging in care (Stengel, 2014, Frazer et al., 2019, Paris et al., 2020). Women also felt that their parenting skills were under scrutiny and that this impeded their ability to receive quality care. This demonstrates a lack of trust and confidence in health care, affecting health care outcomes (Birkhäuer et al., 2017).

To improve the acceptability of care and how care is perceived, health care workers require training on how to reduce stigma and deliver compassionate care (Walter et al., 2017) underpinned by a trauma-informed care model (Covington et al., 2008). Working with pregnant women and new mothers using this model can promote a strong attachment with their babies, it can lead to decreased stress and anxiety, guilt, and an increased sense of safety, as well as greater satisfaction with their experience when using the health care systems (Marcellus, 2014). The use of peer workers may be useful concerning the acceptability of care. Peer workers in health care are becoming increasingly more common. While its long term efficacy is largely unknown, a literature review that examined peer work for people with SUDs found that although more research is needed, the model holds promise (Tracy and Wallace, 2016). Encouraging shared decision-making -regarding treatment choices and allowing for greater autonomy is also important and could lead to greater acceptability of care (Friedrichs et al., 2016).

Availability and accommodation and the ability to reach

Availability and accommodation refer to the fact that health services (either the physical space or those working in health care roles) can be reached both physically and in a timely manner (Levesque et al., 2013). This also relates to workforce attributes such as the presence of the health professional and their qualifications. The ability to reach health care relates to personal mobility, such as availability of transportation, occupational flexibility, and knowledge about health services (Levesque et al., 2013).

This review found a lack of suitable treatment for women and their children, which meant that women did not access care at times. Recommendations to improve this include providing appropriate resources and increased funding for treatment places (Ritter and Stoove, 2016). Lack of availability of SUD treatment is a common issue in Australia and other OECD counties, where it has been found that half of the people seeking AOD treatment are currently unable to access appropriate treatment (Ritter and Stoove, 2016). The investment in SUD treatment benefits both the individual and wider society. It is estimated that for every $1 spent, there is a return to society of $4-$7 which includes reduced drug-related crime, lower criminal justice costs, and theft (NIDA, 2018). Transport to treatment services is also recommended, and can improve treatment retention (Tarasoff et al., 2018, Friedmann et al., 2001), and this should be part of the overall care plan if required (Tarasoff et al., 2018).

Affordability and ability to pay

Affordability reflects the capacity for people to spend resources and time to use appropriate services (Levesque et al., 2013). This includes the direct price of a service and the women's expenses and costs related to loss of income (Levesque et al., 2013). This comprises the ability to pay for health care and the capacity to generate economic resources to pay for health care services. Factors such as poverty or social isolation could restrict the capacity of people to pay for needed care (Levesque et al., 2013).

This review found that financial issues and concerns were barriers to treatment access for some women. This is related to the USA, where most of these studies in this review are from, and there have been changes in health care delivery. Since the Affordable Care Act (AFA) in 2014, SUD treatment has been more accessible (Abraham et al., 2017). Similarly, in Australia, a universal health care system funds substance use treatment programs (Haber and Day, 2014). Unfortunately, affordability does not equate to treatment places, and there are increasing demands for treatment.

SUD treatment should be free or low cost. Ultimately, more treatment places are needed to decrease the 'treatment gap', where more people need care than what is available. Reducing this gap requires multiple approaches, including more access to effective treatment, reducing stigma, training health professionals to recognise addiction, educating of clinicians how to use screening tools as well as how to perform brief interventions (NIDA, 2018), as well as investing in SUD programs.

Appropriateness and the ability to engage.

Appropriateness is the fit between services and a client's needs, treatment timeliness, determining the correct treatment and the interpersonal quality of the services provided (Levesque et al., 2013). The ability to engage with a health care service involves the client's participation in decision-making about treatment and includes health literacy, self-efficacy and self-management (Levesque et al., 2013).

This review found that women felt undermined when they considered that their power had been removed, especially regarding interactions with health care workers that involved caring for their babies. On the other hand, women benefited from learning parenting skills and enjoyed the new knowledge and skills that treatment afforded them. Recommendations are that treatment programs include parenting skills that empower women through the provision of knowledge. Provision of care underpinned by principles of empowerment leads to better health care engagement and women stay in treatment longer (Zand et al., 2017). Significantly, parenting skills can promote more responsiveness parenting and increased levels of physical and verbal engagement with their baby (Solis et al., 2012, Suchman et al., 2006), and importantly, resulting in a more secure infant-mother attachment (Parolin and Simonelli, 2016, Niccols et al., 2012). Programs that include integrated treatment programs with parenting programs can reduce the need for foster care placement and reduce child maltreatment and neglect (Niccols et al., 2012).

Summary

Using the Levesque et al. (2013) framework of health access, this review found various issues that negatively affected health care interactions and access to care and treatment. These findings were primarily focused on the experiences of American women and related to their circumstances and service-level barriers. Suggestions to increase access to care include health literacy and skill-building for women, available and affordable treatments as well as ongoing education for staff who work with clients with complex backgrounds to mitigate the profound impacts of stigma, underpinned by a trauma-informed model of care

CHAPTER THREE: RATIONALE AND STUDY AIMS

Rationale

The background review and the literature review have demonstrated that women with SUDs have multiple unmet medical and social welfare needs. Women, as opposed to men with SUDs, warrant particular attention as they are likely to be the primary carers of their children. Women with SUDs, particularly women who inject drugs, have higher rates of pregnancy, stillborn and sexually transmitted infections than the general population and high rates of mental health conditions (Black and Day, 2016, Haber and Day, 2014). This group of women are also at risk of BBVIs and injecting related harm, including overdose and death (Mathers et al., 2013). Furthermore, these women often have long histories of trauma stemming from adverse childhood experiences (Felitti et al., 1998, Smith et al., 2021). Many women also experience repeated trauma due to high rates of IPV and the removal of children into OOHC. Rates of trauma are even higher for Aboriginal women related to colonisation and transgenerational trauma (Funston, 2016)

Health care interactions between women and health care providers are often negative. Women are met with stigma and discrimination within systems that are supposed to support them. This negativity is frequently compounded by the women's fear of child protection workers and their power to recommend the removal of their children. Because of these experiences, women often disengage from care. However, treatment for women with SUDs who are pregnant women or have children can be beneficial. Tailored and targeted, evidence-based programs can increase treatment retention and reunification rates (Doab et al., 2015).

Being able to engage in care is reliant on the availability of care. However, the background review and the literature review found that there are waiting lists for treatment entry, which is a deterrent, as well as a lack of suitable places for children in treatment with their mothers. The review by Jenner et al. (2014), as identified in the background, provided important insights into the state of treatment for women in NSW. However, as this review was conducted in 2012, an up-to-date review of current services is warranted including service level characteristics.

Overall, there is a lack of research in Australia, particularly from the perspective of women with a history of IDU who are pregnant or are new mothers. There is a need to explore the health and psychosocial needs and experiences of these women. Additionally, this study assists in understanding the health and social care interactions with this cohort of women to identify their needs, values and preferences for care. Including women's voices in planning and evaluating services is central to improving the quality of services and health outcomes and identifying strategies to engage women in health care to improve outcomes for women and their children.

Furthermore, women with a history of IDU have additional needs. They are likely to have other treatable and pressing health issues such as HCV, mental health disorders and the need to access suitable reproductive, sexual and PHC services, and social support. It therefore critical to identify what these specific health needs are and assist women to engage with and prioritise their own health care. As health care service utilisation for PWID are typically low (Haber et al 2009), by identifying this group of women's needs, we can plan for appropriate targeted health interventions that increase their uptake of these interventions.

Aims

This study had three aims. The first was to determine the health and psychosocial needs and experiences of pregnant women and women who have recently given birth and are recent or current IDUs in NSW, Australia. The second aim was to provide important insights into how these women perceive health and social support and their experiences of accessing it and how it may or may not address their health and social needs. The third aim was to examine how service providers can best support, plan and deliver appropriate evidence-based care to meet the needs of these women.

This study aims to contribute to the small but emerging body of evidence around how best to engage with and support pregnant women and new mothers with a history of IDU who may or may not have custody of their children. This includes those women who may not be currently in a situation to be reunited with their children. Recommendations to inform policy and practice to improve the health and social outcomes of these women and their children is provided. This population are some of the most vulnerable individuals within the Australian population. It therefore essential to strive for a model of practice acceptable to this client population.

Research questions

The study aims were to address the following research questions.

For pregnant women and new mothers who inject drugs:

1. What services, including both pregnancy and non-pregnancy services are available?
2. What clinical and care guidelines are available to support this group of women?

3. What are the current health and psychosocial status of these women?

4. What are the health and psychosocial needs and service needs of these women?

5. What are these women's health service experiences and interactions with professionals?

This study was conducted in four phases. Phase 1 will provide a situational analysis and contextual data to the study. This occurred through a service review and a guideline review and addressed question 1 and 2. Phase 2 and Phase 3, addressed questions 3 to 5. During Phase 2, qualitative and quantitative interviews were undertaken with pregnant women and new mothers, and during Phase 3, qualitative interviews were undertaken with health, social care and family and DCJ workers who provide care to this cohort of women. Finally, Phase 4 consisted of the data synthesis and interpretation. Table 1 on the following page describes each question and the data collection requirements for Phase 1 to 3. Further details on data collection tools and interviews and data synthesis and interpretation are provided in chapter 4.

Research framework

The following sections will describe the overarching framework applied to the study. A research framework provides structure, helps formulate relevant research questions, provides structure and insights for the findings (Mills et al., 2010).

Social determinants of health and the socioecological model

The concepts of the social determinants of health and the social-ecological model underpinned the research design, data analysis and interpretation of the findings. The social determinants of health (SDH) refer to the conditions in which we live, grow and work and the effects these have on our health overall (Wilkinson and Marmot, 2003). It is well documented that there are disparities in health outcomes depending on where you live in the world. Health status disparities are apparent within countries and cities, and between countries (Marmot, 2005). For example, in Australia, there is a life expectancy difference of approximately 8 to 10 years between Aboriginal Australians and the rest of the nation (AIHW, 2020b). Many of these life expectancy differences are due to social exclusion, poverty, unequal health conditions, social-economic factors, education, access to health care and an over representation of non-communicable disease and injury (AIHW, 2020b).

Table 1: Research question and data collection methods

Research question: For pregnant women and new mothers who inject drugs:			Data Collection
Phase 1	Qu1	What health services, including both pregnancy and non-pregnancy services are available?	Service review: including internet searches, drug and alcohol directories, NSW and non-Government services directories. Contact will be made with service providers to seek and clarify information
	Qu2	What clinical and care guidelines are available to support pregnant women and their young children with a history of SUD	Guidelines review: The Joanna Briggs Institute, Netting the Evidence, the Cochrane Database and the internet using Google and Google Scholar and hand searching.
Phase 2	Qu3	What is the current health and psychological status of these women?	Interviewer assisted administration of surveys using the following validated tools: Edinburgh Postnatal Depression Scale, Karitane Parenting Confidence Scale (KPCS), Lubben Social Support Scale -6, NSW Domestic Violence screening tool, Brief Child Abuse Potential (BCAP) as well as demographics and other health questions including: BBVI screening, general health overview and Sexual and Reproductive Health questions and substance use
Phase3	Qu4	What are the health and psychosocial needs and service needs of these women?	Semi-structured qualitative interviews with women and their care providers.
	Qu5	What are the health service experiences and interactions of these women?	Semi-structured qualitative interviews with women and their care providers.

The presence of a SUD is often a marker for social and economic disadvantage. This may be early childhood disadvantage, low socioeconomic status, single-parent status or community disadvantage (Spooner and Hetherington, 2004). In turn, the reasons that a person uses drugs may be counter-intuitive in that drug use may be initiated to escape harsh social and economic conditions (which may provide for temporary relief). However, the drug use often makes the situation much worse (Marmot, 2005). Considering this, people with SUDs need support and treatment, but the patterns of social deprivation in which the problems are rooted need to be addressed simultaneously; you cannot address one without addressing the other (Donkin et al., 2018).

Specifically, and concerning substance use, addressing each level of the causal chain, from the causes of disadvantage (for example, low socioeconomic status) to the mediators of disadvantage (for example, lower access to resources) to the impacts of disadvantage (for example, drug dependence) are required. This can include economic and social security, supportive conditions in childhood and adolescence, access to low-cost medical care and treatment (Marmot, 2005).

One framework that conceptualises societal influences on health, is the socioecological model. This model, introduced originally as a conceptual model for understanding human development in the 1970's by Bronfenbrenner (1977), was later formalised as a model from the 1990's onwards which seeks to explore relationships between the individual, their environment and health. The individual is placed at the centre. They are surrounded by levels of influences that can positively or negatively influence health – such as individual lifestyle factors, community influences, living and working conditions, and general social conditions (Krug, 2002, updated 2021, CDC, 2015). See figure 1. This framework, which has been used to understand determinants of substance use (Jalali et al., 2020, Nichols et al., 2021a, Snijder et al., 2021), highlights the complexities of transition at multiple levels and considers how multiple layers of influence intersect to shape a person's health and behaviour.

Figure 1

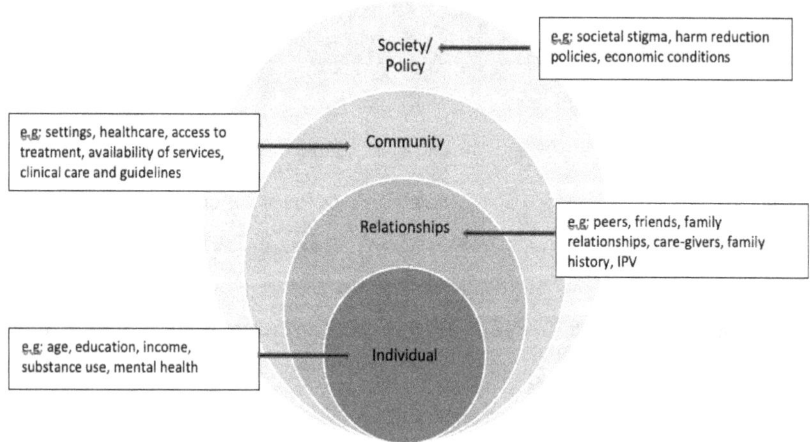

This model and its potential influences on the lives of the women that participated in this research were considered in all aspects of this study. For example, women affected by SUDs and poor mental health are disproportionately affected by domestic violence compared to women without SUD (Brener et al., 2007a). Women were asked about their history of past and current mental health disorders and screened for domestic violence using the NSW Health Domestic Violence Screening Tool (NSW Health, 2006). The role of IPV on women's lives was examined in conjunction with the socioecological model and how this can be addressed across the layers of the socioecological model.

CHAPTER FOUR: METHODS

Mixed methods research

In contemporary health research, several research paradigms exist to search for the truth (for example see (Johnson and Onwuegbuzie, 2004, Ridder, 2014, Osborne, 2008) which is purported as the ultimate goal. Throughout much of the twentieth century, scientific research was mainly quantitative, which originated in science such as physics and chemistry and examined phenomena that could be measured and observed (Tuli, 2010). This type of research requires a reductionist approach focused on numerical values employed to carry out statistical analysis (Gelo et al., 2008). This is known as postpositivist research and relies on logically related steps, deductive reasoning, and control within the research process (Creswell and Plano Clark, 2018).

Over time, social science researchers became dissatisfied with quantitative methods and needed a more in-depth examination of the world within their social contexts (Tuli, 2010). Therefore, some researchers began to undertake their research in more naturalistic settings. This is now commonly known as qualitative research, which draws on the experiences of a relatively small number of individuals' experiences and understandings within their social contexts (Gelo et al., 2008).

Qualitative research takes a constructivist view, where the researcher relies as much as possible on the participant's understanding of the situation as they develop subjective meanings of the phenomena (Creswell et al., 2011). Thus, constructivist research is shaped from individual perspectives and viewed through broad patterns which emerge from the data (Creswell et al., 2011). If we are to view research methodologies on a continuum, we would have postpositivist and constructivist paradigms at opposite ends of the spectrum (Betzner, 2008).

In addition to quantitative and qualitative research methodologies, another research paradigm is mixed methods research. Mixed methods research has been around for several hundreds of years and dates back at least to the time of Galileo in the 1600s, when researchers were using both observational descriptions and quantitative measurements in astrology (Maxwell, 2016). Mixed methods exist somewhere in the middle of both quantitative and qualitative research methodologies and attempt to respect the wisdom of both viewpoints while also seeking a workable middle solution for a problem of interest (Maxwell, 2016). Today, the primary philosophy of mixed methods research is that of pragmatism that attempts to consider multiple viewpoints, perspectives, positions, and standpoints drawing on both qualitative and quantitative research when required to answer research questions (Creswell and Plano Clark, 2018).

Modern mixed methods research in health care and pragmatism as a paradigm

During the 1980s, health care needs and systems were becoming increasingly complex (Greene et al., 1989). As a result, there was a recognition that views from multiple perspectives were required to gain a deeper investigation of complex issues within the health and social environments (Greene et al., 1989). As a result, mixed methods, which takes a pragmatic approach, was identified as a methodology that can bridge the gap between qualitative and quantitative data, enabling participants to voice their experiences (Wisdom et al., 2013).

Mixed methods are important for studies that examine 'human inquiry' (for example, what we do in our day-to-day lives as we interact with our environments), and it allows for knowledge to be viewed as being both constructed and based on experiences (Johnson and Onwuegbuzie, 2004). In addition, it can corroborate findings, minimising the chance of alternative explanations elicited from the data (Shepard et al., 2002). Importantly, for this study, mixed methods research can illuminate phenomena related to vulnerable families, and this would not be captured using a singular approach (Shepard et al., 2002).

Paradigm lens: feminism

As the focus of this doctoral research is focusing on marginalised and vulnerable women, it is vital that this research be viewed through a feminist paradigm that supports empowerment, sensitively uncovers meaning and considers the social, economic and environmental impacts that affect these women's lives (Plummer and Young, 2010). Furthermore, viewing research through a feminist lens allows for a shared set of common epistemological values. These are: valuing women's lived experiences as a legitimate source of knowledge, appreciating the influence of context in the production of knowledge, respecting the role of reflexivity in the research process, rejecting subject-object dualism, and that research can promote social change (Plummer and Young, 2010).

This doctoral research has integrated these values in several ways. This research was conducted by one woman on behalf of the women in the study, a central tenant of feminist research (Hesse-Biber, 2012). Furthermore, women researching on behalf of women is essential when conducting research with women who may be vulnerable or oppressed (Hesse-Biber, 2012).

In line with feminist research, this study also rejects subject-object dualism. Here the researcher's subjective knowledge and experiences are valued and add to the research itself (Plummer and Young, 2010). Research is not viewed as an objective endeavour, and both the researcher and the participants exist in a socially constructed world, and an intersubjective relationship exists between researcher and participant.

The role of reflexivity in feminist research is considered, including examining one's own experiences and their influences on the study (Palaganas et al., 2017, Cook and Fonow, 1986). Cook and Fonow (1986) suggest that reflexivity enables the feminist researcher to include herself in the subject of history so that her perspective develops from her understanding of the situation within the particular context. Reflective practice also promotes transparency within power relations embedded in the researcher–participant relationship (Harding, 1987, Palaganas et al., 2017).

Reflexivity
Reflexivity is an integral part of the research process. Here, the researcher must consider her positioning and different power dynamics that can occur between the researcher and participant (Palaganas et al., 2017), and be aware of how differing values, beliefs, backgrounds, social class, education and perceptions that can alter the construction of reality (Dowling, 2006, Sword, 1999). This view of reflexivity also suggests that engagement with the participant, rather than detachment, which can hinder the research process, is vital for rapport building (Sandelowski, 1986, Palaganas et al., 2017).

I am a PhD researcher and a nurse, requiring that I consider these potentially conflicting roles during this study. According to the International College of Nursing, the nurses' primary professional responsibility is caring and providing professional care, even where a conflict may arise between nursing and research roles (Eide and Kahn, 2008). An example here is when the interviewed women knows that the researcher has professional knowledge and asks for their guidance. This needs to be considered within the ethical boundaries of the research and within the scope of practice of the nurse researcher (Eide and Kahn, 2008). In this study, I was a PhD researcher and not a nurse, and this was discussed within the consent process of the study (Sanjari et al., 2014).

Furthermore, when working with people who may have a history of trauma and substance use histories, there is a risk of vicarious trauma (Branson, 2019). Ways to mitigate this risk for the researcher are through supervision (Branson, 2019). I have access to supervision at work and during supervision with my PhD supervisors. I discussed the interviews with my primary supervisor (without naming anyone or any identifying data). The women that I interviewed were not discussed during my professional supervision, but this may have been helpful considering the populations are similar. I am very experienced in working with and engaging vulnerable groups of women and have worked with this group of women for over 15 years. Before engaging with and interviewing the women, I considered several issues. As a middle class educated white woman, I needed to be cognizant that I would most likely be interviewing women with different backgrounds and histories to my own (Sword, 1999). Being sensitive and compassionate to the information shared during the interviews promotes honesty, reciprocity and trust during the interview process (Davis, 2020). These qualities and attributes are also a part of clinical nursing practice, as required by my professional code 2.2 of communicating effectively and respecting a person's dignity, culture, values, beliefs and rights (NMBA, 2018).

Ways I mitigated some overt differences between the women I interviewed and myself included: dressing casually, being free of expensive branded clothing or jewellery, greeting the women in a friendly manner and introducing myself and thanking them for meeting me (Sword 1999). Straight from the start, I tried to find some common ground. This could be something benign such as the weather or, if appropriate, more intimate details such as having children myself. Pregnancy and birth are unique experiences and can bond women together who have also shared this experience (Savage, 2001). If children were present during the interview, I always engaged with the child in an age-appropriate manner. In addition, I was transparent about my role as a student PhD researcher and a nurse, but my reason for meeting them was as a PhD candidate.

Study design: Mixed methods multi-phase exploratory case study

This study aimed to understand the experiences, health, and social needs of women who are pregnant or new mothers with a recent history of IDU. This required an exploration of the issues that affect these women, including their lived experiences and understanding of their health status (including drug use and mental health history), their social care needs, and their parenting experiences.

This exploration draws upon both constructivist and post-positive epistemologies in a mixed-methods study where both qualitative and quantitative data were collected. Mixed methods is a beneficial methodology for studying social phenomena, as they are often so complex that multiple methods are required (Creswell, 2003). In addition, an exploratory study design is best suited (Fetters et al., 2013), and this has occurred using multiple phases.

Qualitative and quantitative data were collected from the women concurrently, emphasising the qualitative component. These data were rapidly reviewed (Gale et al., 2019) and this informed the qualitative interviews for the health and social care providers and the DCJ workers (Creswell and Plano Clark, 2018). The rapid review which includes the uses of matrices and templates allows the researcher to answer confirmatory and exploratory questions simultaneously while being able to clarify data that may seem contradictory. Qualitative data were then collected from the health and social care providers and the DCJ workers. In addition, women were engaged in follow up interviews, where possible.

The framework applied to this mixed methods exploratory study is a multiple case study approach. Case studies help investigate social phenomena such as experiences and can offer insights into gaps in service delivery (Crowe et al., 2011, Yin, 1999). Case study research involves detailed qualitative and quantitative data collection about the case and is beneficial for exploratory questions (Crowe et al., 2011). A multiple case study approach enables the researcher to draw comparisons within and across cases (Yin, 1999). It has the advantage of using multiple sources of evidence, and multiple realities, offering an opportunity to bridge paradigms (Yin, 1999, Lalor et al., 2013).

The case studies in this study comprise the three cohorts. These are the women, health and social care providers, and DCJ workers. During Phase 2, the first of up to three qualitative and quantitative interviews with each woman took place. Once all recruitment and all primary interviews were complete, the rapid review was undertaken. This informed Phase 3 data collection. During Phase 3 qualitative interviews with health and social care providers and DCJ workers were completed. During this Phase, interviews with women who agreed to a follow up interview and who could be contacted occurred. Finally, during Phase 4, the three cohorts were analysed separately and then interpreted as a final case study. See Diagram 2 of the data collection overview.

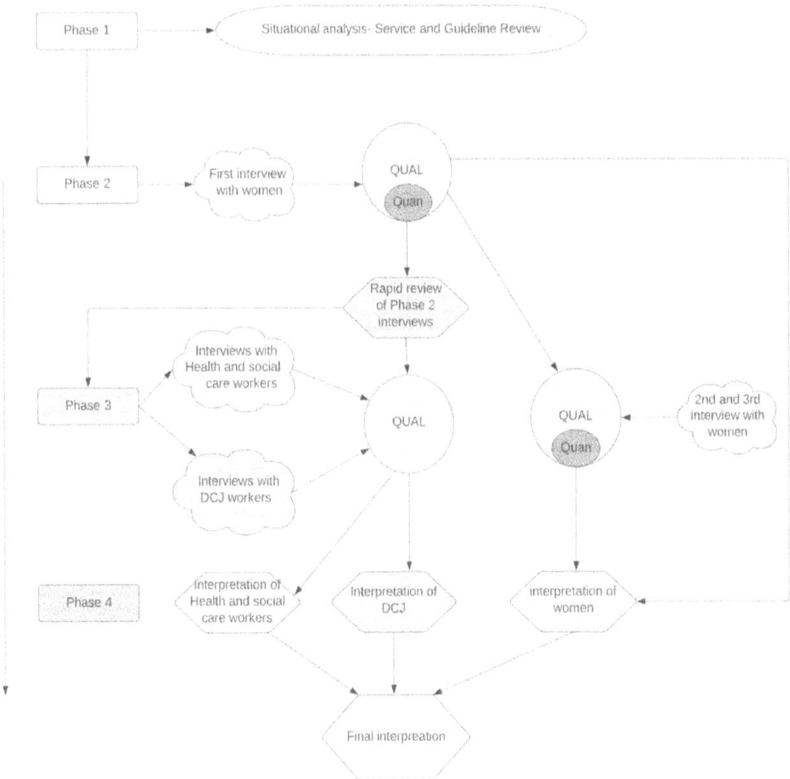

Phase 1: Situational analysis- service and guideline review

This next section describes the methods employed to conduct the situational analysis which consists of the service review and the guideline review. As the research question sought to explore the health and service needs of pregnant women and new mothers who have a substance use disorder, it was necessary to obtain an understanding of the services that exist to support such women as well as the guidelines that are used to provide care for these women. This exploration identified:

- the services available to pregnant and parenting women with SUDs and
- clinical and care guidelines used to direct care for these women.

The service review was conducted in partnership with Kathleen York House. Kathleen York House (KYH), a residential rehabilitation program in Sydney, received a seeding grant from the Community Mental Health Drug and Alcohol Research Network (CMHDARN). CMHDARN is a collaborative project between the Network of Alcohol and other Drugs Agencies (NADA) and the Mental Health Coordinating Council (MHCC), in partnership with the Mental Health Commission of NSW. Kathleen York House received a one off $10000 grant to enhance the research capacity of one staff member who was chosen to receive supervision and support from Professor Angela Dawson. A collaborative project with myself, KYH and Angela Dawson was chosen. The title of the project was: 'A review of evidence to inform substance use disorder (SUD) treatment services for pregnant women'. The aim was to identify best practice guidelines for pregnant women and new mothers who have a history of SUD.

Undertaking this project increased research capacity of the chosen KYH staff member through development of research skills that were acquired by undertaking this project. It also provided groundwork for the service review for Phase 1 of my PhD. The funds were used to release the staff member from KYH four hours a week for the duration of the project so she could undertake supervision and be supported to undertake the project at UTS (See Appendix 4 for the final report). A poster presentation of the findings from the service review were presented at the Australian Professional Society of Alcohol and other Drugs (APSAD) in Auckland 2018 (see appendix 5).

The methods for both the service and the guideline review are described below

Situational analysis: Service review
A mapping method

Methods: In line with the work by Price et al. (2019), a mapping method of health services was employed. A mapping method can help identify services and invite key informants (such as service users or clinicians) to comment on the service. This is usually done through a survey. Price et al. (2019) state that information about services should be freely available to service users, and this mapping can confirm this is the case. The analysis aimed to examine the availability and characteristics of pregnant and parenting with SUD services, the treatment and support provided, and location of these services.

Inclusion criteria: This included current specialist services that provide care to women with SUDs and are pregnant or parenting in NSW. This included both metropolitan and regional areas of NSW and specialist drugs in pregnancy services offered by Local Health Districts and residential rehabilitation settings. Both government and non-government services were included.

The seven-step process as outlined by Price, Janssens et al. (2019) is described as follows:

1. **Defining the target service** – This occurred through systematic mining of grey literature and organisational databases for services that provide care to pregnant women and new mothers with SUDs. This was broadly defined as any service that provided care to women with SUDs in NSW, and these services were found using search engines such as google. Then a systematic approach was undertaken for the review of each database. This included the use of key terms such as 'women', 'mothers', 'treatment' and 'rehabilitation' which were utilised when this was an option. Otherwise, webpages and links associated were systematically reviewed for relevant material.

   Online databases providing information on drug and alcohol services were examined to identify services and the treatment provided, geographical location, cost and if it was a women's only service or not. In addition, NSW Health Local Health Districts (LHD) webpages were reviewed for services that provided specialised pregnancy care in each LHD in NSW.The following databases and web pages were examined

   1. National Drug and Alcohol Services Directory
   2. Australian Drug Information Network
   3. Network of Alcohol and other Drug Agencies
   4. Salvation Army Directory
   5. Alcohol and Drug Information Service
   6. New South Wales User's and Aids Association
   7. Local Health District Government websites

2. **Identifying key informants** – Service managers were identified in step 1 or by contacting the service directly if required.

3. **Data collection** – Service managers were contacted and provided with information about the exercise, its aims and they were invited to participate in the brief survey. Surveys were emailed for completion. Some answers were pre-filled, which was obtained from information that was freely available from the findings in step 1. Service managers were asked to complete the survey and make any corrections as necessary.

4. **The survey** – a brief survey was developed that examined questions such as:
   a) What support and treatment and programs are offered at services in NSW that provide care for such women and their children, and do they follow best practice?

b) What are the aims of these services?

c) Is there a demand for these services (i.e., waiting lists)?

d) How do women access these services (i.e.: referral pathways)?

e) What are the costs to the woman (if any), and how much is this?

f) Are children permitted to accompany their mother, and if so, up until what age?

See Appendix 6 for the full survey

5. **Data analysis** – Data were collated and examined alongside the survey questions. A table was used for the more in-depth analysis of the residential rehabilitation settings. This was guided by the questionnaire that was sent to service providers. Findings were analysed descriptively.

6. **Dissemination of findings** – completed findings were disseminated (with permission) amongst service managers to have an up-to-date overview of other services that provided care to pregnant women and new mothers with SUDs.

Situational analysis: Clinical guideline review

The aim of this review was to examine the quality of clinical guidelines both from Australia and Internationally and to identify their strengths and weaknesses, using up-to-date peer-reviewed evidence and the World Health Organization (WHO) 'Guidelines for the Identification and Management of Substance Use and Substance Use Disorders in Pregnancy' (WHO, 2014) as the 'gold standard'. A clinical guideline provides evidence-based recommendations for doctors, nurses and other health care professionals about the management of care for patients with particular diseases or clinical conditions (Shekelle, 2018). They are informed by a systematic review of evidence and an assessment of the risks versus benefits, and they intend to optimise patient care (Graham et al., 2011).

Data collection for the guideline review occurred through systematic database searches. This included searching for and inputting predetermined search terms as outlined in Table 2 below outlines the databases and search terms used.

Table 2: Database and search terms

Databases used	Search terms
The Joanna Briggs Institute, Netting the Evidence, the Cochrane Database and the internet using Google and Google Scholar as well as hand searching	Substance use/ Substance abuse/ Substance use disorder/Pregnancy/ Perinatal and Clinical Practical Guidelines and Guidelines singularly and in combination.

Only relevant guidelines were examined in detail. These must have met the following criteria: are guidelines for the care of pregnant women and/or women with neonates, AND, substance use in pregnancy, AND, are clinical guidelines for health professionals. Once guidelines were reviewed alongside the WHO guidelines and gaps identified, relevant recommendations were provided, using supporting evidence.

Guideline appraisal

The guideline quality assessment took place using the Appraisal of Guidelines for Research & Evaluation II (AGREE II) Instrument (Brouwers et al., 2010). The AGREE II provides a framework for reaching consensus on methodologic principles and reporting on guidelines that can be used for clinical practice, development protocols, procedural documents and reporting templates (Brouwers et al., 2010). This tool comprises six domains and 23 questions and is designed to assess the quality of health clinical and care guidelines. The six domains are: scope and purpose, stakeholder involvement, rigour of development, clarity of presentation, applicability, and editorial independence (Brouwers et al., 2010). Questions relate to each given domain and are rated according to the statement that it falls under. For example, under domain 1, 'Scope and purpose', the first question is: the overall objective(s) of the guideline is (are) specifically described. The reviewer is asked to rate on a scale of 1-7 how strongly they agree with that statement. Finally, the guideline is scored. See Appendix 7 for the full checklist and the full manual can be found here: https://www.agreetrust.org/

Data extraction and analysis

The WHO Guidelines contain six domains for caring for pregnant women with SUDs, and these formed the framework for the analysis. These domains were summarised, examined and compared using a template (Gale et al., 2019), with guidelines from Australia and other similar OECD countries.

Phase 2 and 3: Interviews with women, health and social care providers and Department of Community and Justice workers

Study participants (cases)
This research applied the term 'case' as defined by Yin, 'An individual person is the case being studied, and the individual is the primary unit of analysis' (Yin, 2014. p31). In this study, cases were women with a history of IDU and their health and psychosocial needs and experiences during the perinatal period. The phenomenon to be explored was not the women as such but their needs and experiences (Baxter and Jack, 2008). To identify the needs and experiences of the final case, a series of interviews were undertaken with three groups. Each of these cases, also defined as a case were: women, health and social care providers and DCJ workers. Findings from these cases informed the final case which was the needs and experiences of women with a history of IDU who are the primary focus of the study.

Case study numbers
While using multiple cases within a case study design is more labour intensive, this design is said to make the overall research more compelling and robust (Yin, 2014). For a multiple case study design, a sampling logic is not required and there are no standardised requirements that state how many cases are needed (Yin, 2014). For this study, the aim was to recruit and follow up to 15 women. In the end, 13 were recruited. For data collection of health and social care workers and the DCJ workers, it was anticipated that due to their workload, the recruitment numbers would be low. Thirteen health and social care workers and six DCJ workers were recruited for one-on-one discussions or as a focus group discussion, depending on workers' preferences and time availability. The interviews sought to establish the health and psychosocial status and needs of pregnant and parenting women with a history of IDU, and their health service experiences and interactions with professionals.

This section outlines the interview process for the women, the health and social care providers and the DCJ workers. See Diagram 3 for the interview schedule. This diagram explains the interview schedule for women during each of the time points. After all the primary interviews were conducted, an initial thematic rapid analysis was conducted. Findings from this analysis informed interviews with health and social care providers and DCJ workers.

Phase 2: Women participants

Thirteen pregnant women and new mothers who were recent or current IDUs were recruited. The aim was to follow them prospectively, starting while they were pregnant and following them up twice postnatally. The time periods for interview were:

- Antenatally 24-to-40 weeks' gestation (time point 0)
- Birth-to-one month postpartum (time point 1)
- Six to nine months postpartum (time point 2).

Participants took part in semi-structured qualitative interviews and quantitative assessments. It was estimated that each interview would take 60-90 minutes. In the end interviews were 45-90 minutes in length and thirteen women were interviewed at various time points. The number of interviews for each woman ranged from one to three. See Chapter 6 for findings.

Diagram 3: Interview schedule

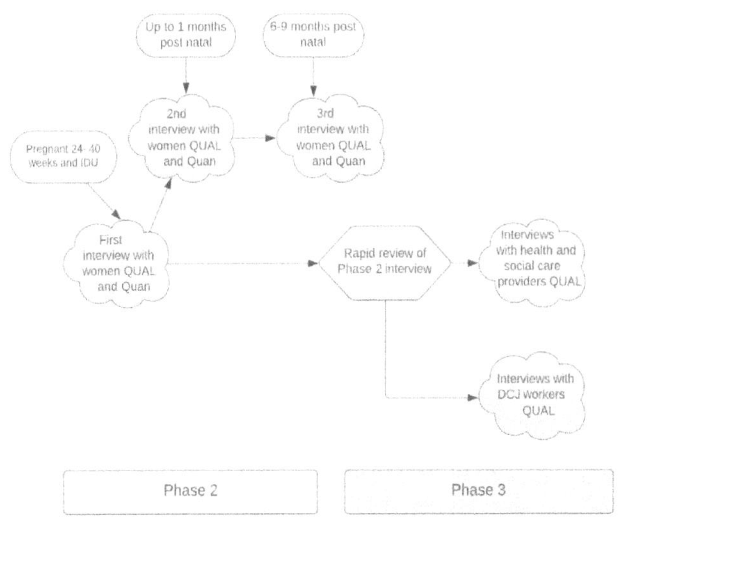

Quantitative assessments

Alongside each of the qualitative interviews, were quantitative assessments. Here, a set of questions that examined demographics and other health questions including: BBVI screening, general health overview and sexual and reproductive health and substance use were asked (See Appendix 8). The following validated tools were utilised: Edinburgh Post Natal Depression Scale (EPDS) (Cox et al., 1987), Lubben Social Network Scale -6 (LSNS) (Lubben et al., 2006), NSW Domestic Violence Screening Tool (DVST) (NSW Health, 2006), Karitane Parenting Confidence Scale (KPCS) (Crncec et al., 2008), and the Brief Child Abuse Potential (BCAP) (Ondersma et al., 2005).

Standardised tools: An overview

This section provides an overview of each of the quantitative measures used.

Mental health assessment tool: Edinburgh Postnatal Depression Scale (EPDS)

Women were assessed for depression using the EPDS (Cox et al., 1987) (see Appendix 9). Scoring was completed after the interview, as per the study protocol. The EPDS allows the researcher to immediately recognise if a woman is at risk of suicidality by a positive score on item 10 of the questionnaire. If positive, this requires immediate action and a referral for mental health support, and this was written into the study protocol (See Appendix 10).

The EPDS is a 10-item self-report scale to screen for postnatal depression in the community. It has been validated and is extensively used in the community and maternity settings. The EPDS has high satisfactory sensitivity and specificity. It was also sensitive to changes in the severity of depression over time. The scale can be completed in about 5 minutes and has a simple scoring method and provided a deeper understanding of the mental health status of the women in the study. Caution needed to be taken with Aboriginal and culturally and linguistically diverse women who may produce lower scores (Austin and Highet, 2017). Scoring occurs as follows:

- Questions 1, 2, & 4 (without an *): Are scored 0, 1, 2 or 3 with top box scored as 0 and the bottom box scored as 3

- Questions 3, 5-10 (marked with an *): Are reverse-scored, with the top box scored as a 3 and the bottom box scored as 0

These are added and a score above 13 indicates that the person is likely to be suffering from a depressive illness of varying severity (Cox et al., 1987).

A score of 0-9 may indicate short-lived symptoms; and 10-12 indicate symptoms of distress that may be discomforting. If the scores increase to above 12, further assessment is required, including a repeat EPDS at a follow up appointment and referral should be considered if indicated depending on the woman's level of distress and social support. A score above 13 requires further assessment, referral and appropriate management is required as the likelihood of depression is high (Austin and Highet, 2017). Item 10: Any woman who scores 1, 2 or 3 on item 10 requires further evaluation before leaving the office to ensure her own safety and that of her baby. This question is related to the risk of self-harm (Cox et al., 1987) No woman scored a positive result on an item, so no referral was required.

Lubben Social Network Scale – 6 (LSNS-6)
This screening tool is validated and provides clinicians and researchers with a self-report measure of engagement with family and friends. It was originally designed as a 12 point scale, and for elderly populations but has since been re-designed and can be used as a six-point scale (Lubben et al., 2006). It has been widely used in many populations, including substance-using populations and younger populations. (Goodhew et al., 2016, Kim et al., 2015). The LSNS-6 total score is an equally weighted sum of six items where each question is scored from 0 to 5. The total score ranges from 0 to 30. The answers are scored: none = 0, one = 1, two = 2, three or four = 3, five thru eight = 4, nine or more = 5. A score of 12 and lower delineates 'at-risk' for social isolation (Lubben et al., 2006) See Appendix 11.

NSW Domestic Violence Screening Tool (DVST)
This tool was used to identify if women were experiencing current domestic violence, within the last 12 months and if they were scared of their current or ex-partner (see Appendix 12). Routine questioning of women about abuse by their intimate partner was introduced in NSW antenatal services, early childhood, drug and alcohol and other drug and mental health services in 2001 (NSW Health, 2006). This was done because of the low identification rates of abuse by health professionals. Data have found that if 10,000 women a month were asked the simple questions presented on this tool, 7.3% of them report experiences of physical abuse or fear caused by their partner or ex-partner within the preceding 12 months (Spangaro, 2007). It is NSW health policy that all women attending the centres as described above are screened for Domestic Violence (NSW Health, 2006).

All women in this study who identified that they had or were experiencing any abuse were to be appropriately referred (see management of DV protocol). Eleven of the women reported recent violence as identified, so the DV protocol was enacted. All women were asked:

    1. Are you safe to go home when you leave here?

2. Would you like some help with this?

All women stated that they had help on hand if required and felt safe.

Karitane Parenting Confidence Scale (KPCS)

The Karitane Parenting Confidence Scale is a self-report questionnaire completed by parents (see Appendix 13). It is used to measure parent's parenting self-efficacy (PSE) (Usui et al., 2020), or confidence in looking after their children aged 0-12 months. It works on a scale in response to a range of questions, using the answers – no hardly ever (0), no, not very often (1), yes, some of the time (2) and yes, most of the time (3). There is the option to answer no, not applicable, which scores (2). There are 15 questions with a maximum score of 30. It has good reliability and validity and was created by a team of researchers at the South Western Sydney Area Health Service in Sydney. It is free to use (Crncec et al., 2008). Each item on the KPCS is scored 0, 1, 2, or 3. There are no reverse-scored items and items have a common scoring order. For each item the first response is scored 0, the second 1, and so on. Items marked not applicable are scored 2. Scores are then summed to give a total score (range = 0-45) (Crncec et al., 2008).

The clinical cut-off for the KPCS is 39 or less. Clients scoring 39 or less are showing clinically significant low levels of parenting confidence. The scoring range is as follows: 40 or more: non-clinical range; score 36-39: mild clinical range; Score of 31-35: moderate clinical range; score of 31 or less: severe clinical range. The reliable change index for the KPCS, is the change in scores necessary for the clinician to be certain that a client has shifted in their level of confidence, is 6 points (Crncec et al., 2008).

Brief Child Abuse Potential (BCAP)

The Child Abuse Potential Inventory (CAP) (Milner et al., 1995) is one of the most widely used and validated measures of child abuse risk (Ondersma et al., 2005). However, the CAP is lengthy and it has 160 items, and can take up to 20 min to complete. Scoring is complex as items are weighted differently (Milner et al., 1995). The Brief Child Abuse Potential (BCAP) Inventory was developed by Ondersma et al. (2005) (see Appendix 14). The BCAP (Ondersma et al., 2005) is a 34-item measure of adult risk for maltreatment of a child. It measures characteristics of the BCAP, that measure risk factors associated with child maltreatment, such as emotional distress, rigidity, and social isolation, rather than asking about abusive behaviours directly. This makes it less vulnerable to socially desirable responses, and more acceptable in various settings. It was initially designed for use as a 33 item measure but an extra question was added after the final paper was published (direct correspondence with author Ondersma 1st February 2017). The BCAP is robust and reliable and correlates significantly with the original CAP (Dawe et al., 2017). It was scored using the scoring template which was purchased directly from the developer. The cut-off score was 12 and above, meaning anyone who scored a 12 or above was at risk of child-abusing their child (Dawe et al., 2017).

Demographical and health data
Demographical and health data examined the following:

- Demographics: age, cultural identity, country of birth, housing, employment status, main source of income, level of education.

- Drug use and treatment: age first started injecting drugs, frequency of drug use, drug of choice, current SUD treatment, history and length of treatment, alcohol and cigarette usage.

- Bloodborne viral infections status: HCV, HBV and HIV status.

- Women's health: Sexual and reproductive health (SRH), including pregnancy history, family planning history, sexual health, and screening history.

- General health status. This was a general question related to other health-related problems such as injecting related injuries, diabetes, heart disease or asthma

Qualitative Interviews
All interviews with women were face to face and completed by myself. The open ended, semi-structured qualitative interviews were recorded, with permission. Field notes were taken to provide context to the collected data. Interviews for the women were one-on-one, and face to face. See Appendix 15 for the interview guides. The interviews were reported using a narrative approach (Fetters et al., 2013). This approach is pertinent to feminist and case study research, where the researcher is engaged in research that explores the experiences of individuals (Fetters et al., 2013). and aims to tell stories of how humans experience the world (Moen, 2006). In addition, a narrative approach is useful for research that is embedded within a social context and seeks to examine and understand how human actions are related to the social context in which they occur and how and where they occur (Moen, 2006).

Justification for the study time-periods
The perinatal period can be a time of heightened vulnerability for women and their babies, that involves significant physiological and psychosocial change and adjustment, including changes in their social status and shifts in power (Eberhard-Gran et al., 2001). The risk is higher again for subgroups of women such as women with a history of SUDs, women with limited social support and histories of trauma and those of low sociodemographic status (Ross and Cindy-Lee, 2009).

This time-period is an ideal time to address substance use and its associated issues among pregnant women as they primarily birth in hospitals (and are therefore more accessible), women may be motivated to change at this point, and there are efficacious SUD treatment programs available for pregnant women. (Ondersma et al., 2014). Considering these factors, the decision was made to attempt to interview women during both the antenatal and the postnatal period to understand their needs and preferences across multiple critical timepoints.

Phase 3: Health and social care providers and Department of Communities and Justice (DCJ) Workers

Qualitative Interviews

Health and social care workers, and DCJ workers who provide care and support to these women were interviewed. Because of the high level of involvement in the care of these women by the health, social and DCJ workers, they were in a good position to be able to add to the overall picture, provide insights into the situation of these women, and to offer advice on how the health and social care gaps and needs can be improved. These semi-structured qualitative interviews occurred once only, which happened in Phase 3. Preliminary data analysis from Phase 2 informed and shaped the questions for these interviews. Invitations were extended to multiple disciplines such as those who provide clinical support (e.g. nurse, midwife or medical doctor) and those who provide social support (e.g. social worker or counsellor) and DCJ workers. Interviewing essential health and social care providers and DCJ workers was important to gain multiple perspectives, insights, and experiences from not only the women themselves but also those involved in their care. Triangulation enhanced and enriched the validity of the data and provided a more complete picture.

Each interview for care providers took 45-60 minutes and were recorded, with permission (see Appendix 16 for the interview guide). Interviews for the health and social care providers were one-on-one, or as a focus group discussion (FGD), depending on their preference and availability.

Fieldnotes

Field notes were kept on each participant, service and experience of conducting interviews with each participant. Notes were descriptive and reflective. Descriptive data included time and date, the physical and social environment, and a brief description of the person who was interviewed. Reflections included my thoughts about the setting, how the interview felt, reflections on the person being interviewed any ideas, questions or concerns that came to mind (Yin, 2014). After each interview, field notes were organised, categorised and electronically stored for retrieval during the analysis phase (Yin, 2014).

Eligibility and recruitment
This section will discuss the eligibility criteria and recruitment procedure for the women, health and social care providers and the DCJ workers.

Eligibility for Women participants
Eligibility for this study was that the women must be pregnant and have a history of IDU in the last six months. All women were required to speak English. Women who would be unable to complete informed consent due to severe mental health issues would not be eligible. See consent form Appendix 17

Recruitment: Women participants
Recruitment occurred through a non-representative purposive sampling technique. This method is beneficial for case studies and qualitative research (Trost, 1986). Cases were recruited from three inner-city Sydney health care facilities, one facility from Western Sydney, and three inner-city rehabilitation centres. Additionally, the women were screened for eligibility to ensure they have a history of recent or current IDU (in the last six months) and could speak English.

Each study site was offered an initial meeting to receive information about the study, including the study aims and methods and the gaps in knowledge. During this meeting, we discussed recruitment, how confidentiality, participant payment and the protocols. In addition, staff had the opportunity to ask questions and clarify any unclear points.

Staff at each study site were crucial to the success of this study. Staff assisted with recruitment and participant follow up, therefore it was essential they felt comfortable with the research and the protocols. Ethics permission was granted for each site.

Recruitment overview:
- Study site personnel were invited to participate in the study.
- Study site staff assisted with identifying eligible women.
- Study site staff explained the context of the study and the study aims to potential study candidates. Consent was obtained from women to be contacted, and they were provided with a study flyer.
- If permission was granted, I contacted the women to arrange an initial meeting.

- I went to the study site (or elsewhere) to further discuss the study with potential participants, obtain informed consent and complete the first interview if appropriate.

- Targeted and multiple contact details using a multidisciplinary team were collected to enhance follow up (Nguyen et al., 2007).

- Consenting participants were reminded that they were free to withdraw from the study at any time without explanation or consequences that would jeopardise their future care.

Eligibility for health and social care participants

All health and social care providers who provided face-to-face care to pregnant women and new mothers with a history of IDU. This includes nurses, midwives, doctors, social workers, counsellors, psychologists and case managers. See consent form Appendix 18.

Recruitment: Health care and social care providers

Eligible staff from the same settings where women were recruited were invited to participate. Staff were contacted directly via email, after being provided with their contact details via a centre manager or nominated contact. Staff were provided with information about the study and its aims. They were allowed to ask questions about the study if they wished.

Recruitment sites

NSW Health Local Health Area Health Services
1. Kirketon Road Centre (KRC) – South Eastern Sydney Local Health District

2. The Langton Centre – South Eastern Sydney Local Health District

3. Royal Prince Alfred Drug Health – Central Sydney Local Health District

4. Drug Health Services – Western Sydney Local Health District.

Non-government organisations (NGO)
1. Jarrah House

2. Phoebe House

3. Kathleen York House

These study sites were chosen as they regularly care for pregnant women and new mothers with a history of drug use and were conveniently located within the inner city of Sydney, or within an area easily accessible within metropolitan Sydney.

The KRC is a PHC centre, in Kings Cross Sydney, providing care and treatment to at-risk young people, sex workers and people who use drugs. It operates under a one-stop-shop model of care, where multiple needs can be met under the one roof. KRC provides an access methadone program and an antenatal clinic for pregnant women.

The Langton Centre is an outpatient clinic located in Surry Hills, Sydney. The centre provides specialist alcohol and other drug treatment services for people who use or are dependent upon alcohol and/or other drugs. It has a specialised chemical use in pregnancy service (CUPS) that offers interventions before, during and after pregnancy to ensure better outcomes for women and families affected by alcohol and other drug use in pregnancy (NSW Health, 2009).

Royal Prince Alfred Drug Health and Perinatal and Family Drug Health (PAFDH) and Drug Health Services at Western Sydney Local Health District have a specific Drugs Use in Pregnancy Service (DUPS). The drug and alcohol focused models of care, with substance use in pregnancy services primarily co-ordinated by drug health services. It is a collaborative model of care, with maternity services tending to take the lead with support from drug and alcohol and other hospital services (NSW Health, 2009).

Jarrah House is an NGO that provides care to pregnant women and new mothers on a ten-week program. Opiate replacement therapy is provided if required. Some women then move on to a longer-term rehabilitation program depending on need.

Phoebe House is an NGO that provides long term on-site residential rehabilitation services offering maintenance OAT for women with or without children for up to nine months.

Kathleen York House is an abstinence-based NGO rehabilitation program in inner-city Sydney, it provides a six-month program for women with SUDs. It does not offer OAT, but children under the age of 12 can stay with their mothers whilst they are in treatment.

Eligibility for Department and Community Justice participants
All DCJ workers who provide face-to-face support and case management for pregnant women and new mothers with a history of IDU. See consent form Appendix 18

Recruitment: Department of Communities and Justice workers
DCJ were approached directly and asked to nominate eligible staff who may be interested in participating in the study. Relevant workers were sent emails and invited to participate. An overview of the study and the study aims were included in the email invitation. They were given the opportunity to ask questions about the study if they wished.

Case study data synthesis and analysis

Definition of case study analysis

Yin (2002) describes data analysis as consisting of 'examining, categorising, tabulating, testing, or otherwise recombining both quantitative and qualitative evidence to address the initial propositions of a study' Yin (2002 p.109). Therefore, this is the method of analysis that is applied to both the quantitative and the qualitative data and the integration of the two forms of data (Onwuegbuzie & Teddlie, 2003).

Data analysis

Data analysis can occur at a single point in mixed methods research, or at multiple points. Once the analysis of the qualitative and quantitative data is complete, combining both forms of data using approaches that mix (or integrate) the data is necessary. This integration is central to mixed methods research and differentiates mixed methods from other types of research and is the point where the qualitative research interfaces with quantitative research (Creswell and Plano Clark, 2018).

Data analysis using a multiple exploratory case design

In this multiple exploratory case design, the primary data collected in Phase 2 informed the data collection in Phase 3, and the integration of data analysis occurred at different points of the exploratory design and then integrated into case studies (Creswell and Plano Clark, 2018).

Phase 2: data rapid analysis

The broad findings of the qualitative and the quantitative interviews with women in Phase 2 informed the research questions for Phase 3. Then interviews were conducted with health and social care providers, and DCJ. Due to time constraints, a pragmatic decision was taken to rapidly analyse the Phase 2 data using a matrix and a template summary (Gale et al., 2019). The use of visual aids such as matrices are useful to summarise data in a systematic, rapid and meaningful way and can be used as a rapid analysis of qualitative data (Gale et al., 2019). The process for the template summary is below.

Rapid analysis: template summaries

Step 1: This involved populating templates with data extracted from the qualitative interview transcripts and the quantitative data into two templates. The first column of both the qualitative and the quantitative data rapid analysis identified key domains based on the qualitative interview guide, and the quantitative questions. The second column in the qualitative data rapid analysis was used to summarise key points from the interviews (Gale et al., 2019) (see Table 3 for the template for the Rapid qualitative appraisal and Appendix 19 for the result). The successive columns in the quantitative data contained findings from each woman interviewed (see Table 4 for the quantitative data template). The findings from this rapid review can be found in the summary table in Chapter 6 (see Table 17: Rapid review and summary of findings).

Table 3: Rapid qualitative appraisal template

Domains	Key points
Overview of pregnancy	
Finding out about being pregnant	
Reaction family/ friends/partner	
Relationship with partner	
Experience with newborns	
Feelings on becoming a mother	
Consideration of own childhood	
Experience with health care providers (midwife, nurse FaCS workers etc)	
How confident are you to care for a newborn?	
Services involved with	
Discussion re: OOHC?	
Requirements to be the best mum	

e appraisal

W1	W2	W3	W4	W5	W6	W7	W8	W9	W10	W11	W12	W

Step 2: Findings from the two template summaries were reviewed alongside the interview questions for the health and social care providers and the DCJ workers (Gale et al., 2019). This allowed preconceived questions to be adjusted to be more focused on the individual needs and outcomes of the women. For example, the women divulged that they had experienced very high rates of IPV. This finding emerged in both data sets and IPV caused physical and mental trauma for women. Therefore, IPV was integrated into the interviews with health and social care providers and DCJ workers in Phase 3. This ensured Phase 3 interviews were informed by knowledge obtained in Phase 2.

The development of themes that emerged during this analysis became building blocks for the in-depth analysis of the final transcripts using Nvivo- 12 software for qualitative analysis. For example, trauma of childing being removed into OOHC was identified in many interview. This became a theme.

Phase 3: data analysis

Qualitative data:
All qualitative data were professionally transcribed verbatim and then checked for any inconsistencies and, or transcription errors. Potential errors were examined alongside the recorded interviews for clarification

Template analysis
A template analysis was used to analyse qualitative data in each of the three data sets. The women, health and social care providers, and the DCJ workers. Template analysis is a structured thematic analysis that involves a hierarchical coding system that is flexible and adaptable to the needs of a specific study (Brooks et al., 2015, King and Brooks, 2018). Additionally, as it is a structured approach to data coding, this enables the provision of an audit trail and a clear demonstration and explanation themes development, for the final thematic structure (King and Brooks, 2018).

Data were analysed using the following method, as devised by Brooks et al. (2015)

1. Initially, each transcript was read and re-read in order to familiarise myself with the data. I also listened to the recordings if necessary, for clarity and accuracy.
2. Key ideas and themes related to the research question were written down and highlighted within the transcripts.

3. Emerging themes were then organised into meaningful clusters, and I began to explore how they were related to each other. This included hierarchical and lateral relationships, as well as narrower themes nested within broader ones.

4. For this stage, the initial coding template on a subset of data began. This was constructed after interviews with five women, six health care workers and three DCJ workers. At this point, several themes reoccurred across the transcripts (see Appendix 20) for the coding templates). The first row contains the highest-order codes that relate to a priori themes from the interviews, and below them are the second-level codes associated with the highest-order codes (King and Brooks, 2018).

5. The themes were transferred to Nvivo 12 software and allocated nodes. This software allows for qualitative data storage, coding, and theme development. This was undertaken by dividing the text into small units (phrases, sentences, or paragraphs), assigning a code label to each unit, and grouping the codes into themes (Creswell and Plano Clark, 2018).

6. The template was finalised and apply it to the full data set. This formed the basis of the findings.

Quantitative data

These data were coded and entered into excel and then analysed descriptively. Frequencies were used to describe the sample's demographics, characteristics, and outcomes as determined by the validated assessment measures. These are the EPDS, the LSNS, the NSW DVST, and the BCAP. As this was a small sample size, generalisability was not attainable.

Phase 4: data synthesis and interpretation

The following section will describe the process of the in-depth data synthesis and analysis of qualitative and quantitative data collected in Phase 2 and the qualitative data collected in Phase 3. Finally, the method employed to synthesise and interpret and all data sets through integration, or mixing of the data, will be discussed.

Final primary data analysis and integration

The mixed-methods design used in this research involved embedding both quantitative and qualitative data into a final case. This design is intended to develop in-depth case studies by integrating multiple data sources. Once the data were analysed separately, it was then analysed at the interpretation stage (O'Cathain et al., 2010). The integration of all data sets, and through triangulation, corroborated findings between data sets to gain a more complete picture of the research questions (O'Cathain et al., 2010). Through this process, a final case was created (Creswell and Plano Clark, 2018).

For this study, data integration occurred at four levels. Firstly, this occurred during the rapid analysis where the broad findings of the qualitative and the quantitative interviews with women in Phase 2 were examined. Secondly, integration occurred at the design level, where results from Phase 2 interviews with women were used to build the Phase 3 research questions. Thirdly, data integration occurred by analysing the qualitative and the quantitative data of the women and integrating and reporting them as one case. Data from interviews with the health and social care providers were and the DCJ workers were integrated as two cases. Finally, data from Phase 1 to 3 were integrated and triangulated during the discussion. Meta-themes were identified at completion of this stage.

The method used to triangulate data is called 'following a thread' (Moran-Ellis et al., 2004). In this method the three qualitative data sets and their thematic findings, the quantitative findings of the women and the service and clinical guideline review, were placed alongside each other conceptually in order to create meta-themes and a broader understanding of the research question (Fetters et al., 2013). Then, based on the literature and the original research questions, a theme in one dataset was chosen; this was from the women's data set as they are the primary focus. This theme was followed across the datasets. Here the idea was to look for patterns or findings or areas of cognitive dissonance, which generated a multi-faceted picture of the issue (Moran-Ellis et al., 2006).

Validating data and rigour

There has been some controversy over the validity and rigour of mixed methods research, and many studies report this very differently, or the qualitative and the qualitative components are reported separately to one another (Brown et al., 2015). According to Yin (2014) mixed methods case study researchers need to examine and consider construct validity, internal validity, external validity (also called transferability in qualitative research Plano Clark and Ivankova (2016) and reliability to ensure rigour. This study, therefore, considered each of these.

Construct validity occurred through triangulation of multiple evidence sources, including the women, health and social care providers, and DCJ workers. This created a multi-faceted view of the situation. Member checking also occurred where transcripts were emailed to DCJ workers for verification and validation. Health and social care providers did not take this opportunity.

Internal validity was maintained by using established analytic techniques such as pattern and thematic matching for the qualitative data analysis. In addition, several of the quantitative tools are validated, meaning that they have been used and validated in other studies and settings, which adds to the overall trustworthiness of the results.

External validity, or transferability. This is a small study and does not claim to be representative. However, as this is a mixed-methods study, and therefore demographical data were collected, as well as standardised tools, and findings may be able to be applied to other similar cohorts of women.

Reliability was enhanced by the use of one person who completed all interviews with all cohorts, therefore reducing multiple researcher bias. Additionally, a protocol was followed for recruitment and interviews, and there was a structured approach to the analysis. Furthermore, integrating data in mixed methods research is important to the overall validity (Zhang and Creswell, 2013). This study mixed data in Phase 2, where the results from the first interviews with women informed the interviews with the other two cohorts. Then again, the data were integrated in stage 4. This occurred systematically using a structured approach that enhanced the overall reliability of the study validity (Zhang and Creswell, 2013).

Ethical issues

This study was conducted in accordance with the National Statement on Ethical Conduct in Human Research guidelines (NHMRC 2015). Prior to participant recruitment, research ethical approval was obtained from the South Eastern Sydney Local Health District Ethics Committee 14/073 (HREC 17/POWH/ 179). Sydney Local Health District and Western Sydney Local Health District provided site-specific approval for the research to be conducted in their districts. The research was ratified by the University of Technology Sydney. The non-government organisations granted approval internally, by their management teams. A separate ethical approval was required for DCJ, which was provided in accordance with their internal processes (Site specific approvals available on request). As this document had 36 pages, only the first and last page are included. The whole document is available on request. See Appendix 21 for the primary and DCJ ethics approvals.

In addition, the National Health and Medical Research Council (2012) guidelines 'Ethical issues into alcohol and other drugs' were examined and used as a framework (Day, 2012). This framework suggested that drug use networks should be consulted when undertaking research with people who use drugs. The NSW Users and Aids Association (NUAA), a NSW users' peer organisation was contacted to ascertain if they would consider involvement in the study processes. Unfortunately, and after multiple contact attempts via email and phone, they were unable to be reached.

Undertaking research with PWID has inherent difficulties due to the illegal nature of illicit drug use, and all care was taken to ensure the participants' confidentiality and all data were de-identified. As the study recruited pregnant women who may also have other children in their care, it was necessary to consider child protection. Therefore, standard child protection notification processes were to be followed if a mother divulged care or behaviour that put their child/ren at risk. This process was described in the consent form and verbally explained as part of the informed consent process.

The Mandatory Reporter Guide (DCJ, 2021b) was to be used if there were potential issues. As part of the consent, it was noted that if there were child protection issues, this would be discussed with the recruiting clinic and the mother. During the interviews, there was no requirement for the Mandatory Reporter Guide to be enacted or child protection issues that needed to be discussed.

Due to the sensitive nature of this study, a protocol for participants who become distressed or upset, or suicidal was developed (see Appendix 22 for the protocol). If this were to occur, they would be referred to an appropriate health professional or the local mental health crisis team. As a nurse with approximately 15 years of clinical experience working with people with SUDs and mental health disorders, I was clinically confident that I could manage these issues if they were to arise. Additionally, the plan was to discuss any child protection issues, or concerns for the mother with my doctoral supervisors. The distress protocol did not need to be enacted.

Confidentiality

All study participants were provided with a pseudonym and their names were replaced in all transcripts. All audio recordings and transcripts were stored on my password-protected computer. Paper copies of the transcripts and consent forms are kept in a secure locked cabinet. Data will be archived at the University of Technology Sydney for seven years after the publication of the report detailing the results. They will be deleted and paper documents shredded according to University of Technology Sydney policy. This procedure adheres to NHMRC guidelines (NHMRC 2015).

Payment of participants

Paying participants for their involvement in research is commonplace and payment for PWID should occur. Payment is for the participant's time and any travel expenses they may have incurred to meet me for the interview. Research has found that offering PWID a modest cash incentive will enhance recruitment and do so, without promoting drug use (Topp et al., 2013). Participants for this study were paid $50 cash per interview, so potentially a total of up to $150 over the course of three interviews.

Conflict of interest

As a nurse working at KRC, there was potential for conflict of interest if I were to personally recruit into the study directly. Therefore, recruitment was undertaken by KRC staff. Staff were responsible for identifying potential participants, and permission was obtained from them for me to contact them directly. At this point, I explained the research, its purpose and aims. I explained that there was no pressure to participate and that they could withdraw at any time without any repercussions

CHAPTER FIVE- PHASE 1: SERVICE AND GUIDELINE REVIEW

Service review

This service review sought to provide an overview of available services in NSW that provide care to pregnant women and new mothers with SUDs. Gaps in service delivery are discussed.

The database search elicited nine in-patient rehabilitation services, two women's day programs and 12 local health district perinatal services. All services were examined; however, the in-patient rehabilitation services were explored in depth. It was anticipated that many women in this study would be accessing these in-patient rehabilitation services or would have accessed these services at some point in the perinatal period and so it was important to gain an understanding of these services and their programs. As outlined in the chapter 1 and 2 of this PhD rehabilitation services hold promise to make positive gains for women and their children. A detailed overview of the database search can be found in Appendix 23. The following services were located during the search:

Public detoxification and rehabilitation programs
1. Guthrie House
2. Jarrah House
3. Kamira
4. Kathleen York House
5. Eloura
6. Phoebe House
7. WHOS New Beginnings
8. Odyssey House
9. Karralika

Day programs and drop in services for women.
1. Dianella cottage
2. Lou's Place

Local Health District perinatal programs
1. Sydney LHD: Drugs in Pregnancy Service
2. South Western Sydney LHD: Perinatal and Family Drug Health
3. Northern Sydney LHD Drug and Alcohol Consultation and Liaison
4. Illawarra Shoalhaven LHD Substance Use in Pregnancy & Parenting Service
5. Western Sydney LHD: Drug Use in Pregnancy Service
6. Mid North Coast LHD: Drug Use in Pregnancy Service
7. Nepean Blue Mountains LHD Substance Use in Pregnancy & Parenting Service
8. Murrumbidgee LHD: Specialist Substance Use in Pregnancy Service
9. Hunter New England LHD: Substance Use in Pregnancy & Parenting Service

10. Central Coast LHD: Substance Use in Pregnancy & Parenting Service
11. South Eastern Sydney LHD: Specialist Substance Use in Pregnancy Service
12. Northern NSW LHD: Drug Use in Pregnancy Service

Western NSW, Far Western NSW and Southern NSW LHDs do not have specialist services.

Summary of findings

Residential rehabilitation services:

Nine services were identified that provide care to women with SUDs who are pregnant and/or caring for young children. Eight of these services are in NSW, and one is in the ACT. The service from the ACT has been included as it also provides treatment to women in NSW. The majority of services are located in Sydney, while three were found in regional areas of NSW. Of the regional services, one is on the Central Coast, approximately 90 minutes north of Sydney, and one in the Blue Mountains, which is approximately one and a half hours from Sydney. The other is in Orange, approximately four hours northwest of Sydney. Except for two, almost all the nine services are women's only services, while the other two provide residential care to single adults and mixed couples. These services are included as they provide care to pregnant or parenting women.

Programs examined run for between six weeks to up to one year. Four programs offer at least a six month program and two programs offer stays for three months and three for stays of between six to ten weeks. Of the nine programs, eight of these programs can have their children in care with them. One program Odyssey House, Sydney, admits pregnant women only until the second trimester. The age at which children can stay in treatment with their mothers varies. Four services take mothers with children up until 12 years old; two will provide care to mothers with children up to eight years, one up to five years of age and one program will provide care to mothers with babies up until one.

All programs provide parenting programs (except this was unknown in one program). Programs offer a variety of parenting programs and include: 1,2,3 Magic, which is an evidence-based child discipline program that allows parents to regain control (AIFS, 2021); Circle of Security which is an attachment-based program designed to increase maternal sensitivity (Cooper et al., 2011); Keys to Interactive Parenting which is an observational instrument designed to assess parent-child interactions during play (Comfort and Gordon, 2006), and Parenting Under Pressure which is also an attachment style programs and has demonstrated benefits for mothers with SUD (Barlow et al., 2013).

Programs for women vary and include a range of psychology based therapies such as cognitive based therapy, dialectical based therapy, motivational interviewing and acceptance, therapeutic community and commitment therapy. Some settings offer interventions such as domestic violence counselling, relapse prevention, anger management, and stress reduction. Many also provide lifestyle programs such as financial planning, cooking, meditation and yoga. A therapeutic community model of practice, a group-based program designed for people with mental health and SUDs, is practiced in three rehabilitation settings.

Two Sydney based services provide OAT on site and one other Sydney based program, and one regional facility provides OAT through a local hospital. All centres charge women a fee for service taken from their social welfare government payment (Centrelink), ranging from 75-80% of weekly pay. This equates to approximately AUD $250-270 a week. In addition, one service requires women to pay an upfront fee and then a weekly price of AUD $20.

Waiting lists were common for these services. Six of the nine services stated that they had waiting lists at the time of asking. One service did not have a waiting list, and this is a specialised service that cared for women on OAT who has been in prison. Waiting lists for two services are unknown.

Centres were staffed with a mix of allied health care workers, which included psychologists, social workers, drug and alcohol workers, counsellors, mental health nurses and nurses. The use of relevant external guidelines was only used within three services. Other services use their own internal policies and engage in quality assurance activities such as client satisfaction surveys. Guidelines used by services were the Drug and Alcohol Treatment Guidelines for Residential Settings, NSW Health (2007) and NSW Health Drug and Alcohol Psychosocial Interventions Professional Practice Guidelines (2008). Both guidelines need updating. One service did not specify the guidelines used.

Some data is missing or unknown. Despite multiple attempts via phone and email over several weeks, three services were unable to be contacted. Therefore, information that was freely available on their websites was used. Additionally, not all questions were always answered for services who completed the short survey (see the summarised findings in Table 5 and the complete overview in Appendix 24).

.

...ential Rehabilitation Services

	KAMIRA	KYH	ELOUERA	NEW BEGINNINGS (WHOS) *	KARRALIKA *	PHOEBE HOUSE	JARR...
	Regional (Central Coast)	Metropolitan	Regional (Orange)	Metropolitan	ACT	Metropolitan	Metr...
	YES	YES	YES	YES	YES	YES	YES
	YES	YES	YES	YES	Mixed	YES	YES
	5-7 months	6 months	6 weeks	90 days	8 weeks	6-8 months	10 w...
...RT	CBT, ACT, DBT	DBT, CBT	X	TC, ACT	TC, SMART recovery	No	Yes, ...
	X	X	X	Yes	X	X	X
	Yes	Yes	Yes	Yes	X	Yes	Yes
	X	X	X	X	X	Yes	X
	Yes	Yes	X	X	X	Yes	Yes
	No	No	No but can facilitate	No	unknown	Yes	Yes
...a	80% of Centrelink	75% of Centrelink	85% of Centrelink and $250 upfront	75% of Centrelink benefit – no money upfront	unknown	unknown	$190... and $... child...
...vices ...DCJ, ...eral	State and Federal funding, Primary Health Network.	Government and donations from private benefactors	State and private funding	State and Federal funding	State and Federal funding and donors	State funding under the (NGO) Program.	State... Fede...
	4-6 weeks	Yes	Yes	Yes	unknown	Yes	Yes, ... wom...
...two	16 women and 6 children.	7 women and 5 children capacity	10 women	24 women	unknown	9 women	24 w... up to...
...ge	Yes	Yes	Yes	Yes, up to the 2nd trimester.	unknown	yes	Yes b... are d... home... last 4...
...ar	Yes, up to the age of 8	Yes, up to the age of 12	Yes, up to the age of 12	no	Yes, up to 12 years of age	Yes up to 5 years	Yes, ... newb...
...ol	NSW Health Drug and Alcohol Psychosocial Interventions Professional Practice Guidelines (2008)	unknown	unknown	unknown	unknown	unknown	NSW guide... other... guide... relev... not s...

| Examines parenting outcomes, drug and alcohol and mental health outcomes, socio/legal/medic al and client satisfaction | Accredited Service- QIC accreditation KPI fixed by the funders and other Quantitative measures | Self-evaluation with a team member/ supervisor | ACHS accredited. | unknown : | unknown | We have internal evaluation systems as as projects conjunctior with universities |

3T: Dialectical behaviour therapy, ACT: acceptance and commitment therapy, MI: Motivational Interviewing, SMART: Self-Management and R
s, ACHS: Australian Council on Health care Standards, QIP: Quality Information Performance Standards.
e

Summary of day programs and drop-in services
The following two services discussed provide day only drop in services for women. These are specific women's only services that provide rehabilitation and programs that allow mothers with children in care to reconnect. Daniella cottage is in the Blue Mountains and Lou's Place is located in inner-city Sydney.

1. Dianella Cottage – A day rehabilitation program for women with a dual diagnosis of mental health and substance abuse issues through trauma-informed care. It does not provide child care but can assist with arranging this service. This service does provide non-residential day rehabilitation assessment, group therapy, assessment, counselling and group workshops, and weekly SMART recovery groups. This program is provided two days per week for seven weeks, during school terms within school hours on Monday and Tuesday from 9.30 am to 2.30 pm. If a woman can afford to pay, there is a $20 fee per group, but this is not compulsory.

2. Lou's place – a daytime refuge for women experiencing trauma, homelessness, domestic violence, mental health or addiction. They provide a program called 'Always Mum' for women with children in out of home care. This program supports women in maintaining contact with their children through measures such as telephone calls and letters. There is no cost to this service, and Lou's place relies on donations and government funding for financial support. They also provide access to basic needs such as food, showers and clothes. In addition, case management and wellness activities are available for women. Their programs underpin empowerment principles and come from a trauma-informed care model.

Summary of Local Health District Services
Of the 15 LHDs in NSW, 12 provide specialist substance use in pregnancy and parenting services (SUPPS). The three LHDs that do not offer a specialist service are geographically situated in regional and remote NSW. The 12 specialist services identified, reported that they provide non-judgemental and supportive care to pregnant women and their families with SUDs. Programs also state that support is provided postnatally but the time point is not specified. Pregnant women are case managed mainly through a Clinical Nurse Consultant and work closely with midwives, doctors, social workers, treatment programs and DCJ workers. The aim is to provide optimal outcomes for both the mother and her baby. These services are government funded, and care is provided through both primary and tertiary health care settings such as community health care settings and hospital based antenatal clinics. These services are free of charge; however, women still need to pay for services

such as transport to treatment centres, and OAT can cost up to around $50 per week, which is expensive for women on social security payments.

Conclusion

Findings indicate a range of services for women in metropolitan Sydney. Services include publicly funded specialist pregnancy services through LHDs, a drop in women's service and six residential rehabilitation services. Services outside of Sydney include one day program and three residential rehabilitation services. There are gaps in service delivery for pregnant women and new mothers with SUD who live in many regional and remote parts of NSW, especially for those living in the Far Western NSW, Western NSW and Southern NSW. There are no specialist services to support women living in these regions who are pregnant and have a SUD. All services are free or low cost.

Two services provided OAT, and two could facilitate OAT through a local provider and waiting lists across all nine residential rehabilitation services can be long. Six of nine services stating they have waiting lists.

Length of treatment times varies and programs that run for at least six months can be a significant predictor for abstinence (Conners et al., 2006, Greenfield et al., 2004). Only four programs provide treatment for six months or more, this may be a contributing factor for women to maintain abstinence once they have left care.

Many if not all (some data is missing) provide attachment-based parenting programs. Attachment-based programs are increasingly recognised as providing a promising framework to develop the mother–child bond, treat maternal addiction and for supporting and promoting a child's socioemotional well-being and attachment security (Parolin and Simonelli, 2016).

Guidelines review

Guidelines for Pregnant Women and New Mothers with SUDs: A National and International Comparison

High-quality, evidence-informed clinical practice guidelines are important to bridge the gap between policy, best practice, local contexts and patient choice, and are an essential part of clinical care (Kredo et al., 2016). This component of Phase1 sought to identify and assess the available guidelines to support pregnant and parenting women with a history of SUD.

Eight guidelines were obtained during the search and these were examined (see Table 6 for the examined guidelines).

Table 6: Summary of examined guidelines

Country	Guideline
Australia	The Australian Clinical Practice Guidelines: Pregnancy Care (Commonwealth of Australia, 2019).
	NSW Clinical Guidelines for The Management of Substance Use During Pregnancy, Birth and the Postnatal Period (NSW Health, 2014).
	Substance Use in Pregnancy. The Royal Australian and New Zealand College of Obstetricians and Gynaecologists (RANZCOG) (RANZCOG, 2018).
	Supporting Pregnant Women Who Use Drugs. A Guide for Primary Health Care Professionals. The National Drug and Alcohol Research Council (NDARC, 2015).
The United Kingdom	Pregnant Women who Misuse Substances, (guideline and interactive pathway) (NICE, 2010, NICE, 2011).
	The Department of Health. Drug Misuse and Dependence UK guidelines on Clinical Management (Department of Health, 2017)
The United States of America	Substance Abuse and Mental Health Services Administration. Clinical Guidance for Treating Pregnant and Parenting Women With Opioid Use Disorder and Their Infants, USA (SAMHSA, 2018b).
Canada:	Substance Use in Pregnancy. The Society of Obstetricians and Gynaecologists, Canada (Ordean et al., 2017).

Each guideline was examined to identify elements related to the six domains outlined in the WHO Guidelines 'Guidelines for identification and management of substance use and substance use disorders in pregnancy' (WHO, 2014).

1. Screening and brief intervention
2. Psychosocial interventions
3. Detoxification
4. Dependence management
5. Infant feeding
6. Management of infant withdrawal

In addition, each guideline was assessed for its quality using the AGREE II instrument (Brouwers et al., 2010). In the following section, each domain will be outlined and its relevance to the international and Australian guidelines will be provided. Identifying any gaps within the guidelines will be discussed.

Domain 1: Screening and brief interventions for hazardous and harmful substance use during pregnancy

Recommendation for practice: Health-care providers should ask all pregnant women about their use of alcohol and other substances (past and present) as early as possible in the pregnancy and at every antenatal visit. Health-care providers should offer a brief intervention to all pregnant women using alcohol or drugs. All guidelines recommended that women should be screened for substance use and that this should be included in the usual antenatal history. This screening should occur at initial assessment (either at time of confirmation of pregnancy, at first booking-in visit, or at first presentation), to ascertain the appropriate model of pregnancy care or provider. This screening should be repeated at periodic re-assessments.

Several guidelines mention the utility of urine drug screens (UDS), whereas the WHO states that self-report screening has been shown to be accurate compared to UDS. Yonkers et al. (2011) found a high degree of agreement between urine toxicology and self-report results for cannabis and cocaine testing in 168 pregnant women. Moreover, self-report was found to lead to more positive reporting of use when a larger window was available for such reporting than was available for toxicology screening, leading to the conclusion that self-report may be a better indicator of use.

The NSW guidelines states that (NSW Health, 2014) pregnant women should have UDS for substance use at the same frequency as non- pregnant women in similar circumstances (e.g., when in an opioid treatment program). The USA recommends that UDS should be used as confirmatory testing, while Canada recommends UDS when clinically indicated. When UDS is clinically indicated this should be performed with informed consent. Pregnant women with problematic drug use should be provided with brief interventions and referred for community resources for further interventions.

All Australian guidelines met these minimum recommendations

Domain 2: Psychosocial interventions for harmful use and dependence on alcohol and other substances in pregnancy

Health-care providers managing pregnant or postpartum women with alcohol or other substance use disorders should offer comprehensive assessment and individualised care. All guidelines recommend tailored psychosocial interventions for pregnant women with SUD when indicated, and that sensitive counselling and referral to an appropriate multidisciplinary drug and alcohol management program should be undertaken.

The NDARC guidelines recommend specific interventions, including motivational interviewing, CBT, counselling, contingency management and relapse prevention. All guidelines except the Canadian guidelines recommend and acknowledge that the staff who will be caring for these women may require additional training, and that care should be delivered in a non-judgmental way and free of stigma.

In addition, the NSW Health guidelines (NSW Health, 2014) and the National Australian guidelines (2019) discuss the need to account for the cultural issues faced by Aboriginal women. They discuss the importance of cultural safety in practice and the differing communities within the Aboriginal and Torres Strait Islander communities and the need to engage with elders as well as Aboriginal health care workers.

Implications for Australia: minimum recommendations met for all Australian guidelines

Domain 3: Detoxification or quitting programs for alcohol and other substance dependence in pregnancy.

At the earliest opportunity health-care providers should, advise pregnant women with SUDS to cease their alcohol or drug use and offer, or refer to, detoxification services under medical supervision where necessary. For women on opioids, they should be encouraged to use OAT whenever available rather than to attempt detoxification. Pregnant women with BZD dependence should undergo a gradual dose reduction, using a long-acting BZD. If a woman develops withdrawal symptoms following the cessation of alcohol, again she should be managed with a long-acting BZD. For women with stimulant dependence, psychopharmacological medications may be useful to assist with symptoms of psychiatric disorders but are not routinely required.

All guidelines have recommendations and treatment guidelines for all substances, in line with the recommendations from the WHO. These are: that pregnant women dependent on alcohol, ATS, cocaine, cannabis, volatile agents, (everything except opioids and BZD), should be advised to cease their alcohol or other substance use, and to do so in a safe and supportive manner. Pregnant women dependent on opioids should be advised to commence on OAT rather than to attempt opioid detoxification. Pregnant women with BZD use disorder should be transferred to a long-acting BZD and undergo a gradual dose reduction. Psychosocial treatment should serve as an integral component of any dose-reduction strategy.

All Australian guidelines met these minimum recommendations

Domain 4: Pharmacological treatment (maintenance and relapse prevention) for alcohol and other substance dependence in pregnancy

Pharmacotherapy is not recommended for routine treatment of dependence on ATS cannabis or cocaine in pregnancy. In addition, the safety of medications for alcohol dependence have not been established in pregnancy, an individual risk benefit analysis should be undertaken on a case by case basis. Pregnant women with OUD should be advised to continue or commence OAT with either methadone or buprenorphine. All guidelines state that there is no pharmacological treatment available for ATS, cannabis, cocaine in pregnant patients. The Australian guidelines mention that nicotine replacement therapy may be relevant if the pregnant woman is unable to quit smoking.

For alcohol use, an individual risk assessment needs to take place and a long acting BZD to be used if necessary. The management of alcohol use and detoxification for pregnant woman and her newborn infant should include supportive care interventions, such as a quiet setting, breastfeeding, cuddling, swaddling, small frequent feeds, and close skin contact (NSW Health, 2014). Pregnant patients with opioid dependence should be advised to continue or commence OAT with either methadone or buprenorphine.

The Australian National guidelines (Department of Health, 2019), and NSW Health guidelines (NSW Health, 2014) specifically mention the needs of Aboriginal women and that knowledge in this area is needed around culture, language and terminology of names for drinking and education around cultural habits and norms.

All Australian guidelines met these minimum recommendations

Domain 5: Breastfeeding and maternal substance use

Mothers with SUDs should be encouraged to breastfeed unless the risks clearly outweigh the benefits. If they are breastfeeding, women should be advised and supported to cease alcohol or drug use; however, substance use is not necessarily a contraindication to breastfeeding. Skin-to-skin contact is important regardless of feeding choice and needs to be actively encouraged. Mothers who are stable on OAT, should be encouraged to breastfeed if it is safe to do so.

The general consensus in all guidelines was that women, including those on OAT should be encouraged to breastfeed, unless the risks outweigh the benefits, such as if the mother is too unstable. Infants with neonatal withdrawal should be offered to be breastfed with support as well as skin to skin contact.

The NSW Health guidelines (NSW Health, 2014), and the Canadian guidelines (Ordean et al., 2017) recommend taking a harm reduction approach, and that women should be informed of the risks and benefits and educated around the safest way to breastfeed. The Australian guidelines do not comment on OAT and breastfeeding, and state that women should not use drugs, including tobacco and alcohol while breastfeeding. The RANZCOG guidelines have little information on the role of breastfeeding and substance use and there is no information on the role of OAT or opiate use for this group of mothers at all.

The UK guidelines (Department of Health, 2017) state that: feeding should be encouraged, even if the mother continues to use drugs, except where she uses cocaine or crack cocaine, or a very high dose of BZD. Specialist advice should be sought if she is HIV positive. The NSW Health (NSW Health, 2014) guidelines recommend that women with HCV and HBV infection can breastfeed, but not women with HIV. This is in line with the WHO guidelines.

Implications for Australia: Minimum recommendations are met for the NSW Health and NRDARC guidelines but not for the RANZCOG guidelines.

Domain 6: Management of infants exposed to alcohol and other psychoactive substances

Health care facilities providing obstetric care should have protocols for identifying, assessing, monitoring and intervening for neonates prenatally exposed to opioids. An opioid should be used as initial treatment for an infant with NAS syndrome if required. If an infant has signs of NAS from withdrawal from sedatives, or alcohol, or the substance the infant was exposed to is unknown, then phenobarbital may be a preferable initial treatment option. All infants born to women with alcohol use disorders should be assessed for signs of foetal alcohol syndrome.

The assessment of guidelines for these recommendations was more difficult. The guidelines recommendation for treating neonates who are, or maybe exposed to substances could not be found for all countries that are included in this synthesis. The intention of the Australian guidelines, the NDARC guidelines, and the NSW Health guidelines is to support the mothers, and so both refer to other guidelines for support related to the management of exposed infants and neonates.

The NSW Health guidelines discuss, in brief the assessment and management of an infant with NAS, and refer to the Neonatal Abstinence Syndrome Guidelines (NSW Health, 2013). These are comprehensive guidelines that discuss in depth the management of NAS, for mothers who use opiates primarily, as well as treatment of non-opiate using mothers with babies who are experiencing a neonatal withdrawal. The recommendations are in line with WHO guidelines.

More up to date Australian guidelines of managing NAS have come from the QLD Government (Queensland Government, 2016). These guidelines provide detailed flow charts regarding the management of NAS, morphine dosing, phenobarbitone dosing and weaning schedules. This guideline also provides a comprehensive list on diagnosing NAS; their list includes suspecting NAS in any baby who is unsettled, is irritable, has a high pitched cry, has tremors or jitteriness, and/or does not feed well and/or has diarrhea.

The USA guidelines (SAMHSA, 2018a) have a comprehensive section that discusses the identification and management of infants with NAS. They recommend the use of toxicology screening although note that this is only beneficial to ascertain recent drug use and it is important to develop a therapeutic relationship with the mother. The NSW Health guidelines also mention this option.

A literature review from Canada that focused on the management of ATS NAS, found that there was no relevant literature regarding clinical effectiveness of interventions for diagnosis or treatment of neonatal abstinence syndrome due to crystal methamphetamine (Wells C et al., 2017).

Implications for Australia: Minimum recommendations met for all Australian guidelines.

Recommendations, additional information and areas for review

Stigma training should be implemented and additional training to meet the diverse needs of women with SUDS. Culturally safe practice is required when supporting Aboriginal women and this is an additional recommendation. Breastfeeding is missing from the national Australian guidelines and there is limited information in the RANZCOG guidelines. This is not in line with WHO recommendations and should be included.

Other areas that are important to mention in the care of pregnant women with SUDS that are mentioned in the WHO guidelines are: comprehensive continuity of care, sleeping practices, mental health, sudden infant death syndrome (SIDS) and tobacco, contraception, trauma informed care, intimate partner violence, and stigma. The following table represents whether or not these issues are included in the following Australian guidelines (see below Table 7: Guideline recommendations)

Table 7: Guideline recommendations

WHO guidelines	Australian	NSW Health	NDARC	RANZCOG
Comprehensive continuity of care	√	√	√	√
Sleeping practices	√	√	√	X
Mental health	√	√	√	√
SIDS and tobacco	√	√	√	√
Contraception	X	√	√	X
Trauma informed care	√	X	X	X
Intimate partner violence	√	√	√	X
Stigma	√	√	√	X

The WHO guidelines recommend a women-centred, trauma informed program to care for mothers with SUDs (WHO, 2014), however only the Australian National guidelines recommended this indicating a gap in the guidelines from NSW Health, NDARC and from the RANZCOG. The Australian, and the RANZCOG guidelines did not discuss the need to include conversations about contraception with pregnant women, and furthermore, the RANZCOG guidelines did not discuss the need to address sleeping practices, IPV or stigma.

AGREE II review

For this PhD the AGREE II tool was used was used to identify the quality of the reviewed guidelines. This was conducted after the guidelines were located. After review, all guidelines were recommended to be useful. Guidelines from the UK, UK (NICE), NSW, the USA and the Canadian guidelines were all strongly recommended as they had domain scores of at least 60% in a minimum of four of six domains (Brosseau et al., 2014, Yan et al., 2013). These guidelines were clear and comprehensive, met many of the criteria presented in the AGREE II tool such as being clear about stakeholder involvement, and were rigorous in their development. The guidelines that were recommended, but required some edits, were the Australian, RANZCOG and the NDARC guidelines. This was because mostly domain scores were between 30% and 60%, or there were some domains that had insufficient or were lacking information (Yan et al., 2013).

A lower percentage on some domains were for reasons such as lacking voices of peers, limited information on editorial independence and at times it was not clear what methods were used to search for evidence. Additionally, limitations were not discussed or lacked clarity around the links between evidence and practice. However, scores are not always indicative of the usefulness of the guideline and guidelines that are more narrow in scope may not describe all the features in the instrument. Further detail is provided in Table 8: Agree II Appraisal. This table provided obtained scores on each domain and its overall recommendation.

al

	D4	D5	D6	Overall quality (out of 7)	Recommend	Recommendations
%	61%	38%	0%	4	Yes, with edits	Despite not scoring high on many of the domains here, these are simple ¦ Suggestions: to take a harm reduction approach in regards to breast feec to include contraception as post pregnancy discussion and referral. Lacke stakeholders and peers. Little or no information about editorial independ
%	83%	54%	83%	6	Strongly recommended	Inclusion of trauma informed care would strengthen this otherwise very ¦
%	88%	20%	41%	5	Yes, with edits	Does not mention UDS but as this is performed in General Practice this sh limitations. The need to account for cultural issues faced by Aboriginal we is little information on the role of breastfeeding and substance use and t¦ role of OAT or opiate use for this group of mothers. Sleeping practice, coi informed care should be discussed. Contraception is very pertinent to GF peers.
%	83%	45%	0%	4	Yes, with edits	It would be helpful if the information about its development was include¦ and easy to read, with clear instructions for use. The GL could be improve work from a trauma informed care perspective. Lacked information abou or no information about editorial independence
%	83%	71%	81%	5	Strongly recommended	Clear and easy to use. Good suggestions for follow up of women, maintai instructions for women experiencing IPV. There is not a lot of informatioi guidelines or if key stakeholders were utilised. Good information around women about CPS and guilt. Lacked information about stakeholders and
%	88%	90%	91%	6	Strongly recommended	These are very clear and comprehensive GL that include perspectives of ¦ professionals. An abridged version would be helpful as this is over 300 pa
%	83%	71%	91%	6	Strongly recommended	These are very clear and comprehensive GL. It provides working example Includes a comprehensive section that discusses the identification and m¦ This is helpful to have in the same GL
%	88%	71%	91%	7	Strongly recommended	Clear and comprehensive GL. Provides information on UDS, harm reducti breastfeeding and comprehensive care. Limitations and alternative treati

Guideline summary

Using the WHO guidelines as a gold standard reference point, the minimum recommendations are met for all International and Australian guidelines for domains 1, 2, 3 and 4. However, the Australian National guidelines and the NSW Health guidelines mention that culturally appropriate care as additional consideration for domains 2 and 4. In regards to domain 5, the recommendations are met for the Australian, NSW Health and NRDARC guidelines however the RANZCOG guidelines have little information on the role of breastfeeding and substance use and there is no information on the role of OAT or opiate use. A risk versus benefit view should be undertaken for breastfeeding and OAT should be recommended when clinically indicated. The recommendations for domain 6 were met however, the information was fragmented, difficult to find and needs updating.

Additional information found during the analysis identified that the WHO guidelines recommend women-centred, trauma care for mothers with SUDs. Only the Australian National guidelines recommended these additional approaches. Additional information on contraception needs to be included in the Australian National guidelines and the RANZCOG guidelines, and the RANZCOG guidelines should add in discussions on sleeping practices, IPV and stigma.

Considering the strengths and limitations of each guideline as previously described, and outcome of the scores using the AGREE II tool, and the comparison to the WHO and the international guidelines, the Australian guideline that is most applicable, comprehensive and user friendly is the NSW clinical guidelines for the management of substance use during pregnancy, birth and the postnatal period (2014), and will be referred in the discussion section of this thesis. If required, and others will be referenced as needed, especially where gaps exist in this guideline for example the need to include trauma informed care.

Finally, the RANZCOG guideline, with extra inclusions, has the potential to improve the lives of pregnant women with SUDs significantly. While there are many specialised services for pregnant women with SUDs, as described in the service review, many women may choose antenatal provided through a GP, especially if they do not divulge drug use. This is known in NSW as a 'shared care' approach where the antenatal is provided by a GP and a hospital setting (Charlton et al., 2015). Therefore, the inclusion of cultural competent care for Aboriginal women, sleeping practices, contraception and trauma informed care can benefit these groups of women. Additionally, the role of role of breastfeeding and substance use and OAT needs to be included as a best practice option for mothers who use opiates and will benefit mothers who divulge substance use in pregnancy in general practice settings.

CHAPTER SIX- PHASE 2: OVERVIEW OF WOMEN AND QUANTITATIVE FINDINGS

Rapport building and establishing trust were key elements to this study for women to feel comfortable sharing their experiences. Women mostly spoke very candidly about their experiences, frustrations and difficulties, and what it was like to be a mother with a SUD. While there did not appear to be any engagement issues, I took my cues from women's body language, expressions and tone. I offered them a break or the opportunity to speak at another time if required. This was not necessary. I felt honoured to be a part of this research and the recipient of such rich and deep data. Several of the women thanked me for the opportunity to tell their stories and said they were discussing issues that they had not spoken to anyone about before. This, and the willingness of women to talk, and many agreeing to a follow up interview, reassured me that the study was worthwhile, important and of benefit to interviewed women. Firstly, an overview of the interviewed women will be described, followed by the quantitative findings.

Overview of women

Thirteen women were interviewed between August 2017 and May 2019. Interviews took place in parks, rehabilitation centres, street benches, and one woman was interviewed in my car as I drove her to her rehabilitation graduation ceremony. Primary interviews occurred at various stages ranging from four months gestation to eleven months post-partum. Three women were interviewed during pregnancy, and the rest were interviewed postnatally. Of the 13 women, the majority (7/13) were interviewed once, two women were interviewed twice, and three women participated in three interviews. The interviewing schedule is on the following page in Table 9. All women provided written consent and were allocated pseudonyms. Interviews were recorded with permission, and women were provided with $50 cash.

Table 9: Interviewing schedule

Woman no#	Pseudonym	Initial interview	Follow up interview 1	Follow up interview 2
1	Veronica	4 months pregnant	5 weeks post-partum	not interviewed
2	Diana	8 months pregnant	5 weeks post-partum	not interviewed
3	Natalie	8 months pregnant	not interviewed	not interviewed
4	Samara	8 weeks post-partum	7 months post-partum	8.5 post-partum
5	Heather	4 weeks post-partum	not interviewed	not interviewed
6	Cathy	5 weeks post-partum	not interviewed	not interviewed
7	Alannah	5 weeks post-partum	not interviewed	not interviewed
8	Ash	6 weeks post-partum	6 months post-partum	13 months post-partum
9	Jo	2 months post-partum	not interviewed	not interviewed
10	Faith	6 months post-partum	not interviewed	Not interviewed
11	Izzy	9 months post-partum	not interviewed	not interviewed
12	Ella	10 months post-partum	17 months post-partum	20 months post-partum
13	Nicola	11 months post-partum	not interviewed	not interviewed

Demographics of women

At recruitment, women were aged between 27-40 years of age, and their cultural backgrounds and identities varied. Five of the 13 women identified as Caucasian, five women identified as Aboriginal, two women identified as Asian and one woman as Persian. One woman in the cohort had completed tertiary education, and five women had completed 12 years of schooling. Five women had completed less than ten years of education. Of the women who had not completed ten years of education, all women identified as Aboriginal. The majority of the women (9/13) stated that they were in a de-facto relationship at the initial interview, while the remainder were single.

All women were reliant on social welfare for income. Six women received a Newstart payment, six received a Parenting payment, and one woman was on a disability support payment. Housing stability was an issue for almost half of the women. At the time of the interview, six women had no fixed address. Of these six women, three women were housed in a short-term rehabilitation centre, two women were housed in a long-term rehabilitation centre, and one woman was living in a hostel. Seven women had secured long-term housing, with six women obtaining a Department of Housing tenancy, and one woman had her own private accommodation. Several women had transient housing experiences throughout their pregnancy and four women had lived on the street at some point and one woman had also 'couch surfed' while she was in her final trimester of pregnancy. Almost all women (12/13) had entered a rehabilitation centre during their pregnancy, and two women were incarcerated whilst they were pregnant (see Table 10: Demographics table).

Table 10: Demographics table

n = 13 woman	
Age (median)	33.5 years (range: 27-40 years)
Ethnicity	
Caucasian	5
Aboriginal*	5
Asian	2
Middle Eastern	1
Main source of income	
Parenting payment	6
Newstart	6
Disability support payment	1
Highest school level completed	
Tertiary	1
Higher school certificate (year 12)	5
Year 10	2
Less than 10 years of schooling	5
Relationship status	
De-facto (none were married)	9
Single	4
Accommodation type at time of interview	
Department of housing	6
Tertiary homelessness -housed in a short term rehabilitation (but no fixed address)	3
Tertiary homelessness -housed in a long term rehabilitation (but no fixed address)	2
Tertiary homelessness-housed in temporary hostel (but no fixed address)	1
Own private housing	1
Other types of accommodation while pregnant**	
Primary homelessness (lived on the street)	4
Tertiary homelessness (couch-surfing)	1
Incarceration	2

*All identified as Aboriginal and *not* Aboriginal and/or Torres Strait Islander
** Does not add up to 13 as not all women had experienced these types of accommodation

Quantitative Findings of Phase 2 Interviews with Women

This section provides an overview of the quantitative findings from interviews with women. The findings presented here are from the first interview, and if data are shown from any of the follow up interviews, this will be specified. An overview and summary of all quantitative findings used for the rapid review is located at the end of this chapter (see Table 16: Rapid review and summary of findings).

nd treatment histories

bes substance women used in the three months preceding the primary interview. This is represented in Table 11 an

ed in the perinatal period

m	Pregnancy / post-natal stage	Injecting drug use in the three months preceding interview 1				Other substances used	
		Heroin	CMA	Cocaine	Fentanyl	THC	Tobacco
	4 months pregnant	2-3 times weekly	no	no	no	no	no
	8 months pregnant	daily until seven months pregnant	no	no	no	no	daily
	8 months pregnant	no	daily	no	no	no	daily
	8 weeks post-partum	daily until delivery	no	no	no	no	daily
	4 weeks post-partum	daily until 8 months pregnant	no	no	no	weekly	daily
	5 weeks post-partum	no	daily until delivery	no	no	daily	daily
	5 weeks post-partum	once when pregnant	Once when pregnant	no	no	daily	daily
	6 weeks post-partum	once while pregnant	no	no	no	weekly	daily
	2 months post-partum	daily until 8 months pregnant	no	no	no	no	daily
	6 months post-partum	two to three times weekly	no	no	Daily for one month	daily	no
	9 months post-partum	once to twice weekly	2-3 times weekly	no	no	no	daily
	10 months post-partum	2-3 times weekly	no	no	no	no	daily
	11 months post-partum	2-3 times in the last three months	weekly for 2 months	no	no	no	daily

hetamine. BZN- Benzodiazepine. THC- Tetrahydrocannabinol. ETOH- ethyl alcohol.

Most of the women interviewed for this study had engaged in frequent substance use in the preceding three months of the interview (see Table 11: Substance use and frequency), and the majority of women (11/13) were injecting drugs at least weekly. Six women were injecting daily. Almost all women (11/13) were daily cigarette smokers; however, none of the women drank alcohol. Two women used BZD during their pregnancy (valium) in addition to heroin, and this BZD was used weekly. Women commonly consumed marijuana, and almost half (6/13) used this in addition to other substances in the perinatal period.

Heroin was the most commonly injected drug for this group of women. Over half (8/13) reported heroin as their primary drug. Four of the women were using heroin daily almost up until the birth of their babies. Two women had also used BZD weekly, and one of these women had smoked until she entered rehabilitation. Another woman who was four months pregnant used heroin two-three times per week. This was her only drug used and she did not smoke tobacco.

Two other women had relapsed and started using heroin two to three times a week when their babies were six and eleven months old. One of these women also smoked tobacco daily, and the other woman had been using fentanyl patches when she found it hard to get heroin and smoke THC daily. One woman who was five weeks post-partum when interviewed had used heroin once and CMA once in the last three months in pregnancy. She smoked cannabis and tobacco daily. A different woman had used heroin once in the preceding three months during her pregnancy. She was a daily smoker and used cannabis weekly before her baby was born.

Of the women who reported CMA as their primary drug, one woman who was five weeks post-partum at interview, was using CMA, cannabis and tobacco daily, until she birthed her baby. Another woman who was interviewed when her baby was 11 months, had been using CMA weekly for two months until she went into rehabilitation. Before entering rehabilitation, she used heroin two to three times in the last three months and was a daily smoker. A different woman who was a daily smoker had relapsed in the community and used CMA two to three times a week over two months before entering rehabilitation. She had also used heroin once to twice weekly during this relapse period. Her baby was nine months old when she was interviewed.

Finally, a woman who was interviewed in the community when she was eight months pregnant was using CMA daily and smoking tobacco daily and BZD weekly (valium). She was admitted to a rehabilitation centre as soon as she had her baby at full term.

Substance use treatment: Pharmacological treatment

Pharmacological treatment for heroin use played an important role in these women's lives, with eleven of the 13 women interviewed on OAT at the time of interview. Opiate agonist therapy was not indicated for the two remaining women, as they used CMA. Of the 11 women who were on an OAT program, they had all been on OAT in the past. In addition, as nearly all women had used heroin during their pregnancy, 11 of the 13 children were prescribed morphine for NAS at birth.

Mental health

Table 12: Mental health history

Mental health history	Number of women
Self- reported mental health disorder	12
On psychiatric medication	7
Edinburgh Depression Postnatal Scale (interview 1)	
0-9 (may be some mild distress that is short lived)	6
10-12 (may be some distress that is of discomfort)	4
>12 (the likelihood of depression is high)	2
>18 (the likelihood of depression is very high	1
Positive score item 10 (requires immediate evaluation to assess for harm to self and/ or baby)	0

Almost all women (12/13) stated that they have histories of past or current depression and or anxiety. Only one woman stated that she did not have a history of past or current mental health history, but scored a 10 (above normal range) on the Edinburgh Depression Postnatal Scale (EDPS) (Cox et al., 1987).

According to the cut off criteria for the EDPS, at least two women could be diagnosed with major depression and four with minor depression (Cox et al., 1987). Four women scored in the 10-12 range, which may indicate the presence of symptoms of distress that can cause discomfort. Two women scored in the high range, above 12 and one woman scoring a very high 18 which signifies that the likelihood of depression is high. No woman scored a positive score on item 10 (indicating immediate risk of suicide) (See Table 12: Mental health history).

Just over half of the women (7/13) interviewed for this study were prescribed psychiatric medications, and additionally, two other women had been on psychiatric medication in the past but were not taking these medications at the time of the interview. Six women were prescribed an antidepressant medication, and one woman was taking antipsychotic medication.

Blood Borne Viral history

Five women reported that they were HCV PCR positive, one woman had HBV in addition to HCV. One of these women with HCV was commencing treatment in the rehabilitation centre where she was residing.

Sexual and reproductive health care

Antenatal screening and sexual and reproductive health care

Just over one third (4/13) of women attended antenatal screening on time (before ten weeks of pregnancy) (DoH, 2016). Four women attended their first antenatal appointment at 10-20 weeks, and five women attended the first appointment when they were over 20 weeks pregnant. Reasons for late presentation for antenatal screening included not knowing they were pregnant, fear of child removal, unstable substance use, and denial of the current pregnancy. One woman who presented very late for her first visit, at 32 weeks, said that she knew from quite early in the pregnancy that she was pregnant but was in a state of denial and was fearful that her baby would be removed from her care the moment it was born.

Two women stated that if they could have easily accessed an abortion early on in their pregnancy, they would have considered this an option. One woman attempted to access post-coital emergency contraception, but the pharmacy was shut. This woman also stated that she would have considered a termination but it was between Christmas and New Year; while she had felt this was an option, she thought that this service would be unavailable. Another woman who considered termination an option was living in a small regional town and was unsure how to access this service.

Contraception and cervical screening

Ten of the 13 women were interviewed postnatally and none had commenced using any form of contraception. Nearly all (12/13) women stated they had been offered contraception at the hospital post-partum and were referred to their GP for follow up but this did not happen. Some women commented that they did want contraception but had not 'got around to it', or they did not feel that they needed contraception as they were no longer in a relationship. The local hospital proactively followed up one woman who had seven children and they encouraged her to have a tubal ligation. She was considering this. Another woman was considering the contraceptive implant 'Implanon' when she was interviewed.

Over half of the women (7/13) said that their cervical screen was up to date. Two women said that they had been screened for sexually transmitted in the previous twelve months

Children and out of home care

Number of children per mother (n=47 children).

Table 13: Out of home care

Number of children per women*	
One child	2 women
Two children	4 women
Three children	1 woman
Four children	1 woman
Five children	2 women
Six children	1 woman
Seven children	2 women

*This does not include the child of the women who was only interviewed once while pregnant as it is not known what happened to them postnatally

Amongst the 13 mothers there was a total of 47 children. Most women, (11/13), interviewed had previous children. Two women had one child only, four women had two, one woman had three children, one woman had four children and five women had five or more children. The ages of the children ranged from newborn up to 22 years of age (see Table 13: Out of home care).

DCJ and Out of Home Care

Of the 11 mothers with previous children, ten mothers had children in OOHC. There were 35 out of a total of 47 children living in OOHC with the majority of the children in care with other family members. Of the 11 women with children in OOHC, all children lived with their grandmothers or close family. Maternal grandmothers play a prominent role in caring for their daughter's children. Five grandmothers had one child each, one grandmother had three of her daughter's children, another grandmother had responsibility for four children, and one grandmother cared for five children.

At the time of interview, one of the 11 women interviewed had care of her older children. Her children were girls aged 11 and 13. This mother said that there was no ongoing DCJ case for either of these girls and that she had the support of her partner, who was the father of her newborn infant but who was not the father of her daughters.

Validated tools

The following section describes the findings from the validated tools that were completed during the quantitative interviews

Lubben Social Network Scale

Table 14: Social support scores

LSNS Scores	n=13		
	Family subscale (out of 15)	**Friends subscale** (out of 15)**	**Total scores (out of 30)**
High scores 6-15	5 women	2 women	13 - 30 = 1 women
Low scores <6	8 women	11 women	<12 = 12 women

According to the Lubben Social Network Scale-6, scores from six of the 13 women indicated that they had marginal family ties, and nearly all women, 12 out of the 13 indicated that they had marginal friendship ties. Twelve out of the 13 women were at risk for social isolation. This includes the overall score of both the family and the friendship subscale (see table 14: Social support scores)

Of the five women who indicated they have some support from family, four were Aboriginal and they indicated they had strong ties to their mothers, cousins and siblings. Only two of the women overall indicated that they had more than one friend whom they could call on for support in times of need, talked to at least once a month, or felt at ease with. Of these women, one woman was an Aboriginal woman who had strong ties to her 'street' community, and the other woman had established friends who she had known from some time. She was living in a rented house through the Department of Housing in the community with her two older children aged 11 and 14.

Parenting confidence

Table 15: Karitane Parenting Confidence Scale

Karitane Parenting Confidence Scale (KPCS) *	Number of women
Score 40 or above (confident)	10
Score of 39 (mild low parenting confidence)	1
Score of 36 (moderate parenting low confidence)	1
Score of 30 (severe low parenting confidence)	1

*Mothers scoring 39 or less may be experiencing low levels of parenting confidence

Most women scored high on the parenting confidence scale with ten out of the 13 women scoring confidence in caring for their newborn infants. Of the woman who achieved a low score of 30, she was living in a rehabilitation at the time of the interview and did not have her child in her care. This woman was interviewed twice more and her KPCS score increased to 39 on subsequent interviews. She did not have her child in her care at the follow up visits. The woman who scored 36 had her older two girls living in her care and was pregnant at the time of interview. She was subsequently interviewed, this time with her newborn in her care. Her score increased to 39 at the follow up interview. The woman who scored 39 on interview one lived in a rehabilitation centre with her young son, and she was a first-time Aboriginal mother. This is the only time she was interviewed. Of the women who were interviewed more than once, none of their scores decreased (see Table 15: Karitane Parenting Confidence Scale).

Brief Child Abuse Potential (BCAP)

Table 16: Brief Child Abuse Potential Scores

Mother	Pseudonym	Perinatal stage	BCAP - Interview 1	Perinatal stage	BCAP Interview 2	Perinatal stage	BCAP- Interview 3
1	Veronica	4 months pregnant	Low risk	5 weeks post-partum	Low risk	not interviewed	nil
2	Diana	8 months pregnant	Low risk	5 weeks post-partum	**High risk**	not interviewed	nil
3	Natalie	8 months pregnant	**High risk**	not interviewed	nil	not interviewed	nil
4	Samara	8 weeks post-partum	Low risk	7 months post-partum	**High risk**	8.5 months post-partum	**High risk**
5	Heather	4 weeks post-partum	**High risk**	not interviewed	nil	not interviewed	nil
6	Cathy	5 weeks post-partum	**High risk**	not interviewed	nil	not interviewed	nil
7	Alannah	5 weeks post-partum	Low risk	not interviewed	nil	not interviewed	nil
8	Ash	6 weeks post-partum	**High risk**	6 months post-partum	Low risk	13 months post-partum	Low risk
9	Jo	2 months post-partum	Low risk	not interviewed	nil	not interviewed	nil
10	Hope	6 months post-partum	Low risk	not interviewed	nil	not interviewed	nil
11	Izzy	9 months post-partum	Low risk	not interviewed	nil	not interviewed	nil
12	Ella	10 months post-partum	Low risk	17 months post-partum	Low risk	20 months post-partum	Low risk
13	Nicola	11 months post-partum	Low risk	not interviewed	nil	not interviewed	nil

At the primary interview, four women were categorised as at high risk for child abuse of their children when assessed using the BCAP. One woman who was interviewed once when pregnant, was admitted to a long-term rehabilitation after her baby was born, and the outcome for her and her baby is unknown. Another woman who was initially interviewed in a rehabilitation setting, was then discharged home into the community with her baby. She was re-interviewed twice and each time was categorised as low risk for child abuse. At the first interview, two other women were also categorised as at high risk for physical abuse. One of these women did not have her baby in her care at the time and she self-discharged from the rehabilitation while her baby was in DCJ care. The other woman who had her baby in her care at the interview, was involuntarily discharged from the rehabilitation setting back into the community with her baby. Despite multiple attempts at follow up, the outcomes for these two women are unknown.

A different woman, was categorised as at low risk for child abuse at the first interview, was then categorised as at high risk for the subsequent two interviews. She did not have her baby in her care at any of the interview time points. Contact was inadvertently made with this woman six months after her last interview, when I saw her at my place of work, and her baby was now living with her grandmother in another state (see Table 16: Brief Child Abuse Potential Scores).

Intimate partner violence

According to the NSW Health DVST, violence was an issue in at least nine women's lives. However, the qualitative interviews, suggested the level of violence in these women's lives was more pervasive, where 12 of the 13 women divulged that IPV was an issue. Of the women who stated that IPV was an issue using the DVST, five women stated they were afraid of their partners. All these five women were receiving IPV support and training through the rehabilitation centre that they were staying at, at the time of interview.

Not all women divulged the type of violence that was occurring however, some mentioned intimidation, physical and psychological violence and threats of self-harm, if they were to leave. Two women described having been assaulted so badly that they were hospitalised. One woman had a broken jaw and was beaten repeatedly to the head so severely that she now suffers from epileptic seizures. Another woman had been assaulted so many times by her ex-partner that she has arthritis in both her arms and legs.

uantitative appraisal and quantitative findings summary	Diana	Natalie	Samara	Heather	Cathy	Alannah	Ash	Jo	Hope	Izzy
a	Diana	Natalie	Samara	Heather	Cathy	Alannah	Ash	Jo	Hope	Izzy
0	Tertiary	HSC	HSC	Year 10	< year 10	HSC	HSC	HSC	<yr 10	<yr 10
an / an	Caucasian Australian	Caucasian Australian	Persian Australian	Caucasian Australian	Aboriginal	Aboriginal	Asian Australian	Asian Australian	Aboriginal	Aboriginal
	De-facto	De-facto	De-facto	De-facto	De-Facto	De-Facto	De-Facto	De-Facto	De-Facto	Single
	DoH	Rehab	Rehab	Rehab street	Rehab	Rehab	Rehab and DoH	DoH	Hostel Street, rehab	DoH rehab street
ther	In rehab with mother	DCJ	In rehab with mother	DCJ	In rehab with mother	In rehab with mother	In rehab with mother	Baby in her care	DCJ	In rehab with mother
with	Yes, x 3 with grand-mother	Yes, x 1 with grand-mother	Yes, x 1 with grand-mother	Yes, x 4 with grand-mother	Yes, x 4 with grand-mother	Yes x 1-DCJ	Yes x 1 with grand-mother	Yes x 2 with grand-mother	no	no
	yes	yes	no	yes	yes	yes	yes	yes	yes	yes
	On time	On time	10- 20 weeks	10- 20 weeks	> 20 weeks	10- 20 weeks	> 20 weeks	> 20 weeks	> 20 weeks	10- 20 weeks
	Yes	Yes	Yes	Yes	Yes	Yes	Yes	Yes	Yes	Yes
t	Pregnant	pregnant	Nil	Nil	Nil	Nil	Nil	Nil	Nil	Nil
	HCV	Nil	HCV	Nil	HCV	Nil	Nil	Nil	Nil	Nil
	Yes	Yes	Yes	Yes	Yes	no	Yes	Yes	Yes	Yes
	Yes	Yes	Yes	Yes	no	Yes	Yes	No	No	no
	0	8	3	0	12	9	10	9	12	6
	5 15 X	19 X X	9 12 13	14 X X	12 X X	5 X X	15 9 7	7 X X	4 X X	7 X X
	14 12 X	12 X X	10 11 11	2 X X	6 X X	5 X X	10 11 11	12 X X	5 X X	6 X X
	40 40 X	30 X X	42 41 42	44 X X	43 X X	41 X X	40 40 41	36 X X	45 X X	41 X X

Summary of findings

A diverse range of women were interviewed for this study. Five women were Aboriginal, five Caucasian Australian, two women were Asian Australian, and one woman was Persian. All interviewed women were reliant on government payments for income, they nearly all had transient and unstable housing with many living in a rehabilitation service at the time of interview, not knowing where they were going to live once discharged. Four women lived on the street at some point during their pregnancy or once their baby was removed and they had left rehabilitation. Women experienced high levels of IPV and nearly all had histories of mental health. Five women had self-reported HCV and one HBV. None of the eligible women were on contraception.

Nine women were on OAT, and over half of women were at risk of social isolation. At the primary interview, four women obtained scores which suggests that there was potential for child abuse. Eleven women had previous children, and ten of these women's children were in OOHC. Mostly women felt that they were confident parenting their newborn. Substance use levels were high and although no tool was undertaken to ascertain levels of addiction, use was very high in a subset of women with six women injecting heroin or CMA daily. These findings indicate that women are extremely vulnerable, and at increased risk for overdose, bloodborne viral infections, homelessness and issues related to IPV and further pregnancy. In addition, the limited support that many women have, along with high rates of self-reported mental health histories paints a picture of extreme marginalisation.

CHAPTER SEVEN: PHASE 2 QUALITATIVE FINDINGS OF WOMEN

This chapter describes the findings of the 13 women who generously gave their time to share their experiences with me. The aim was to provide women with a voice and an opportunity to discuss their needs and experiences and how they perceived care provision during the perinatal period.

This section describes the findings from the qualitative interviews with 13 women. It includes data from the primary interview, and follow up interviews with five of the women. The seven themes identified within the data were: abandoned and alone, power(less) and in the dark, constant surveillance and the burden of proof, trauma and child removal, sadness and guilt, catch 22- being set up to fail and desire for a normal life.

Theme 1: Abandoned and alone

The women discussed feeling let down and abandoned by the health and social care systems that are there to support them. The women noted that they were provided with many resources while they were pregnant and in the immediate post-natal period. However, some women stated that the high level of support provided initially tapered off after the birth of their babies. For example, one woman (Ash) described that she was in active addiction after having her baby removed at birth, and she felt that no one cared. She was on a methadone program but said that she did not always turn up for her daily dose and nobody checked in on her. Simultaneously, she was experiencing IPV and reported that her partner regularly removed her mobile phone. Ash acknowledged that this may have affected services from contacting her, and so she felt alone.

> *Um, I really didn't feel I had much support after that, the DCJ worker called me and said, "look, you know, you need to get into a rehabilitation"... but like I thought I was pretty much on my own afterwards. I had domestic violence issues, and my partner would take my phone away from me.* Ash interview 1

The considerable support Ash received when she was pregnant had ceased; once she gave birth and her baby was removed into OOHC, it wasn't about her anymore, and she felt alone, with minimal resources or support. Ash was no longer a priority for the health care providers.

> *'Yeah...the doctors no longer were looking after me. And then, when they passed me to another bunch of doctors, and there was a lack of communication. I felt like that no one worried about me as such....'* Ash interview 1

When Ash was asked at which point she felt that she was not supported, she stated the following:

> *About three days after the caesarean, I think maybe because they felt that I didn't really need to be there anymore... Maybe because I was in high risk [ward] and so*

> *I had all these nurses* [and then]*, I wasn't high risk anymore* [as her baby was no
> longer in her care]*…. And didn't need to have the same level of care anymore.*
> Ash interview 1

Another woman also experienced this lack of ongoing support from care providers. Veronica was 14
weeks pregnant when she was first interviewed. She was on a buprenorphine program through a
local pharmacy. Veronica found it surprising that if she missed a dose of her buprenorphine, she was
not followed up.

> *'And I missed a day at the pharmacy* [buprenorphine] *because I wasn't feeling
> well… and nobody said anything. I thought they'd be really on my case. But
> nothing. So yeah. I don't know really where I can turn to'* Veronica interview 1

Veronica felt isolated during her pregnancy due to service changes. She said that she preferred the
support at the public OAT clinic where she had received treatment, before being dosed at the
community pharmacy. At the time of the interview, she was waiting for the chemical use in
pregnancy service to contact her. Waiting for this appointment caused her anxiety. Veronica stated
she was using heroin heavily in the early stages of her pregnancy (five days a week) but wanted to
do the 'right thing'. She had started to decrease her drug use but needed further support to reduce
this further.

> *And I just noticed now that I'm going to the pharmacy. I feel like there's no
> support at all…You know, when you're at the clinic* [the OAT clinic]*, I kind of felt
> there was support there. There's help there, but now that I'm at the pharmacy,
> I'm thinking, I could really be mucking up here, and no one will know.* Veronica
> interview 1

Izzy described a similar scenario. She had a six-month baby boy in her care when she transferred
from a public OAT program to a community pharmacy prescriber. Izzy felt more isolated when she
began picking up her methadone from the pharmacy and became more withdrawn. She gradually
started missing more and more methadone doses and then used heroin. Izzy felt that if she had
been given the opportunity to stay engaged with the local substance use in pregnancy team and had
remained with the OAT team at the public clinic, she might have avoided a relapse and not have had
her son removed.

> *Interviewer: 'So, what support do you think you needed at that point to keep you,
> safer and not using'?*

> *Izzy: If I kept going back to* [the substance use in pregnancy team], *and picking up*
> [my methadone]*…but I moved a chemist because I was doing good… I thought,
> "Yeah. I'm all right. You know, I'll pay for a chemist". That's when it started up and
> missed my dose and then I just kept going to get on* [use drugs]. Izzy Interview *1*

The findings of the interview data analysis indicate that some women felt abandoned by their DCJ workers and health care workers when their cases had been closed. This may have occurred because they were deemed to be doing well, leaving women vulnerable to substance misuse, compounded by poverty. Izzy, who had her case closed, wanted DCJ to remain in her life, but as she was, according to her, doing well and therefore no longer needed the extra support. She was looking after her one year old boy for six months in the community, on her own, with very little social support. Izzy described being short of money, so she began dealing drugs to provide her with extra income. She thought she could stave off the temptation to use. One day she said she thought, 'I can have a little bit', and she ended up relapsing. When asked about what support she was provided with from DCJ during the six months before she relapsed, Izzy replied 'none' and she felt cut off from them.

> *'Like um, yeah, when they just cut me off…DCJ, like they shut my case, so there was no involvement with them'.* Izzy Interview.

Nicola shared a similar story to Izzy and started selling and using drugs after her DCJ file closed and support ceased. When I met Nicola, she was homeless, living in a rehabilitation facility with her one-year-old girl, and afraid of her violent partner. Nicola has a complex and long history with DCJ. She has five older children in DCJ care and living with her mother in another state. She has been allocated two different DCJ workers on two separate occasions to support her and her one year old. Both times the cases have been closed. The first time her case was closed, Nicola started selling drugs as she needed the money. She then began injecting heroin and subsequently was told that she needed to go into rehabilitation immediately or she would lose custody of her child.

> *'They closed the file after three months, then they walked back into my life a couple of months ago and said, 'You have to either leave with your kid* [and enter treatment], *or we're taking him'.* Nicola Interview 1

Since this time, Nicola has been staying in the rehabilitation and says that she is nervous as her case is due to be closed again. Nicola was worried that without ongoing support from her DCJ worker, she would lose this child to DCJ care. In addition to the substance use, Nicola was concerned about the IPV from her partner, which was ongoing before she entered the rehabilitation centre.

> *So, um, then I wasn't in danger* [as I was in rehab], *so they could close my file. They were in that much of a hurry to close my file that they didn't think about what they were doing to us, you know?... Yeah, and they've closed my file now and left me with it. Do you know what I mean?* Nicola Interview 1

Nicola explained that she felt abandoned by her DCJ worker and left to sort out everything independently. She needed assistance with ongoing issues related to her ex-partner, including a long history of violence, unstable housing and financial issues. These issues are described in the following comment:

> *'He's like, "Oh, you're doing so well. See ya"' Sign me off, but he's left me with to solve all the problems by myself…Whereas everyone else has got a DoCS worker to support them…You know, and financial help and stuff. I don't have anything'.* Nicola Interview 1

Another woman, Faith, said that she wished that her case had not been closed, as she felt that the provision of care through DCJ would keep her accountable, more connected to services, and off drugs.

> *Yeah, but I did want them there because that was sort of uh--something to pull me up…To scare me into not using…Yeah, keep me in line, and then they sort of just didn't care, so I just sort of didn't care, and I thought I was on my own, so yeah. I started using again, like selling and then using.* Faith Interview 1

Faith felt that she needed DCJ overseeing her care to provide some boundaries, but she was left with none when her case was closed.

> *And then, like, yeah, to leave a place like this and have some support like, DoCS sometimes close your case when you do what they want you to do, so that's what happened with me last time, and then I had nothing. So, you know? No boundaries, nothing.* Faith Interview 1

Faith, who was interviewed whilst she was in rehabilitation for the second time and had been allocated a new DCJ worker for this occasion, found it unusual that she had no contact with her DCJ worker during her stay. She felt that it would have been better if there had been some ongoing contact so she would not think she was on her own.

> *'I've had no contact with DCJ since I've been here- I don't know what they're doing with me, and they, you know? Just don't have any contact with them. So, I don't know what's going on. I'm just here'.* Faith Interview 1

Women described experiencing regular intimate IPV. The trauma related to this violence and the removal of their children was magnified when there was very little or inadequate support in place. This heightens their feelings of being alone and raises their levels of fear and anxiety.

Five women stated that they were frightened of their partners or ex-partners and had to live wondering where they were, and for those male partners who were incarcerated, when they would be released and what this would mean for their safety. In addition, these women felt that they had to deal with this situation on their own, with little or no support, and that this lack of support from services meant that they feared the IPV would resurge again, and they felt unsafe.

One woman stated that if her ex-partner is released from prison and approaches her, she will need to take an apprehended violence order (AVO) out on him to keep her and her baby safe.

> *'If he comes near me, I'm just gonna put an AVO on him…you know my baby needs to be safe'* Faith Interview 1

However, the women noted that AVOs are not a guarantee of safety and that they would have to deal with their violent ex-partners breaching these orders independently. Veronica had experienced the failings in this system first-hand. She had taken many AVOs out against her ex-partner in the past but commented that the response from the local police had been relatively poor, and they were judgemental.

> *'it's disgusting, and they just don't get it…because I've had a few with attitude towards me and I just think 'wow''* Veronica Interview 1

Her ex-partner kept breaching the AVOs, which meant she lived in fear. Veronica commented that some police officers do not take IPV seriously, and she did not trust them to keep her safe. Another woman felt that her partner was left with no help and the police provided insufficient support regarding the IPV he inflicted on her. She was left with no choice but to keep away from him. When asked what would have been helpful for her partner at this time, she said it if they had *'told him how to go about mending his family or go and get help'. Heather Interview 1*

Nicola considered that there was no actual violence as it was not physical, but she had been informed by DCJ that there was violence and that if she wanted a chance to keep her baby, she had to leave. However, her partner would not allow her to go when she tried to escape. Eventually, she did leave but was annoyed that he had not been provided with any support around managing his IPV. This lack of support meant there was no chance of them remaining as a family.

> *'Yeah. That's it, I couldn't take him* [the baby] *to a safe place, but the thing was that… He wouldn't let us leave, but at the same time, once they got us out, they didn't tell him how to fix it. You know what I mean? So it was a real catch 22 there'.* Nicola Interview 1

Cathy described receiving little support when her children were removed in the context of IPV. She used drugs as a 'crutch' to cope with the trauma of having her children taken into OOHC and felt that she may have reacted differently if she had been provided with support during this difficult time.

> *Like they didn't help me get out of that relationship. I was in a violent relationship for ten years, and it's not as easy as they think...You know what I mean? Like, they've got to help the mother. They took my life when they took my kids. Like, I just didn't see the point in giving up the drugs or, you know what I mean? Like actually I was hardly on drugs, I was stepping away. I never had touched the ice, um, until they were ripped.* Cathy Interview 1

The feeling of being abandoned was again identified as an issue by one mother who described a time when she was pregnant for the third time and she said that she had 'fallen to pieces' when her daughter was removed. She described how this experience had a lasting impact on her and that she felt that she was left alone and with no support at all.

> *'I fell to absolute pieces, and my fiancé, who I thought had my back, didn't, he got in gaol; I was just standing there with nobody. No family, no friends, nobody'.* Natalie Interview 1

Theme 2: Power (less) and in the dark

It was evident that some women had very little control over certain aspects of their lives that they found distressing. For example, others often made decisions concerning custody of their children, the placement of their children into OOHC, and decisions regarding access to rehabilitation. The women were also unaware of decisions made and provided with little information concerning such processes. As a result, the women felt frustrated and powerless as they could not participate in making decisions that directly affected them.

Cathy, who had a long history of IPV, had one of her children removed from her at birth. She felt that the process, and how she could aim for restoration was not adequately explained to her in a way that she understood. At the point when DCJ removed her child, Cathy was asked to sign some legal documents. Cathy is illiterate and although she said she was provided with a verbal explanation, she felt this was not sufficient and was unsure what she was signing.

> *'None of them read it to me.. They just explained that's what, and I'm like, 'Okay. So I have to sign the paper'. I didn't realise what I was actually signing'* Cathy Interview 1

This situation signifies the power differences between care providers and these women, especially for women in vulnerable situations and with low literacy levels.

Power in the form of violence was common. Women had experienced a range of violence, including verbal intimidation and restrictions of freedom, which included preventing them from leaving the house, withholding contact with anyone outside the home, and removing mobile phones. Women were also physically assaulted, which resulted in hospitalisation for two women. Cathy stated that she has ongoing medical issues related to a violent assault by her ex-male partner and she had required hospitalised.

> *'I fought so hard and then uh,...and he bashed me again, really badly, and nearly killed me. That's why I've epilepsy now...I had a seizure while I was giving birth to him'.* Cathy Interview 1

Diana explicitly discussed the power imbalances that she felt existed between her and her DCJ worker. When Diana was interviewed for a second time, she was very frustrated that she had no clear plan for her future. She felt that others had power over her life. Diana demonstrates this feeling through the following quote.

> *They've got the power... I feel like they want me to jump through hoops; there are other cases here* [at the rehabilitation] *where they help them, they give them a time frame to go home...but I'm the only one that feels like my life's a mess. I don't know where I'm going, and it's scary because I have a baby.* Diana Interview 2

Faith also spoke explicitly about the differing power roles between her and her DCJ worker. Because of this power in-balance, she felt that she did not want to open up to her worker, as she would just be told what to do with minimal consultation. Faith did not like discussing concerns with someone she felt had power over her. She said:

> *Somebody who thinks that, because I have power over you, and then I can sort of tell you what to do, and they talk to you as if they're telling you what to do. And I don't like that, so I don't open up to people like that... so I have had no contact with DCJ since I have been here* [in the rehabilitation]. Faith Interview 1

Two mothers described their experiences of being 'in the dark'. This concerned health professionals and DCJ workers who knew that they were going to have their children removed within days of giving birth, but they were not told until the last minute. These women wished that they had been provided with more information leading up to the birth of their children, and that if this had occurred, outcomes could have been different.

Heather was in short-term rehabilitation when I met her, and she had her child removed from her care within days of birth. Heather said that she was completely unaware of the DCJ decision to remove her baby into OOHC and that she only realised at the last minute.

> *'You know what I mean? And that was the thing. Like, um, nobody told me*
> *anything. I just would … I knew that I had to do perinatal meetings, but there was*
> *just, there was no clarity. There really wasn't'* Heather Interview 1

Heather was asked how she felt about this when she said the following.

> *'And that made it difficult, and that made it more uncertain for me, so as soon as*
> *DCJ came into the picture* [at the hospital], *I didn't know what was about to*
> *happen except they were there to take my child'.* Heather Interview 1

Similarly, a different woman spoke about her experience of child removal and that she was unaware, until the end, that this would occur. Samara has been using heroin throughout her pregnancy; she was homeless at times and experiencing violence from her partner. She was on a methadone program for the last four months of her pregnancy, where she received intermittent antenatal care. Samara was not aware that she was going to have her baby removed at birth:

> *'No, I didn't know until like, right at the end when it hit me. Um, because it was*
> *like, yeah, they said, oh yeah, he's going into care now. You can't have him back'.*
> Samara Interview 1

Samara stated that she was not sure why her son had been removed but would have liked to have had a chance, to work with DCJ and keep her son. Samara said she had not been informed there was a risk her son would be removed if she did not work with DCJ. If she had known, she may have made contact with DCJ sooner and engaged in more timely antenatal care.

> *'Not really… but I wanted to know my options, you know what I mean'* Samara
> Interview 1

During the third interview, Samara became increasingly frustrated with her interactions with DCJ workers and described the continued feeling of being powerless, like she was a puppet on a string.

> *'Everyone like pulling strings for you. Like a puppet…I don't know I'm get to pee*
> *by myself. I have to pee on cue'* Samara Interview 3

Alannah was interviewed postnatally in an inner-city park. She had lost custody of her newborn within days of giving birth. She described how she felt that she was left in a hopeless situation in general; and powerless to make her own decisions about her care. In addition, she had been in gaol for several months during her pregnancy. When asked what support she was provided with when she was released from prison, she replied:

> *'What do they help with, darling? What throw you out in the paddock with*
> *nothing to fucking do?'* Alannah Interview 1

She was discharged from prison, whilst still pregnant, into a Western Sydney women's refuge. However, this was not her preferred option, and her request for rehabilitation was ignored.

> *'They could've got me into rehabilitation while I was in fucking gaol like I asked the cunts'.* Alannah Interview 1

Alannah was upset about having to go to gaol when she was pregnant and felt that if she was allowed to go to rehabilitation instead of prison, she would have been able to keep her child. When I asked Alannah if being in gaol provided her with housing security at the time, as she was pregnant and homeless, she replied:

> *'What do you mean? I'd rather be without a roof than fucking be there...Like, what can you fucking do in there?...At least if I'd got to rehab, I would've got shit sorted and then I... would still have my fucking child'* Alannah Interview 1

During her pregnancy, Alannah had a difficult time. This was complicated by disengagement from health and social care services. One day she threatened a staff member from the hospital during an antenatal appointment where she was due to have an obstetric ultrasound. She described being overwhelmed by the number of people in the room, and she became upset with the staff attempting to do her ultrasound. Alannah had been raped when she was 14 years of age and found having to undress in front of people for medical care challenges. The following comment represents Alannah's distress and disempowerment over the sensitive situation that she found herself in.

> [There were] *too many people in a room, and they just think it's okay. They can have seven or eight of them...that's intimidating. I don't like it. That's when she went to do the ultrasound fucking grab, pulled my pants down, and everyone's seeing my vagina. I got embarrassed. That's why I said, 'Fuck off. I should punch you out.* Alannah Interview 1

Alannah lost custody of her baby girl straight from the hospital and had no contact with her daughter when I interviewed her when her baby was nine weeks old. Alannah was living in temporary accommodation, however, she rarely stayed there, preferring to stay with an older male friend who she said looked after her. She had very little other support and was upset with some of the services that had provided support to her during her pregnancy. She felt that her concerns were often ignored and so just disengaged from health and social care services altogether.

Izzy who also had her child removed, had started using illicit substances again when her baby was around ten months of age. She was informed by DCJ that they were going to take her baby, for his safety. She said she pleaded with them to allow her to get help and go into a rehabilitation setting with him, but they said no.

*Yeah. And then it was just weird because I've, I've done everything for him, and at
18 months down, they just come take him to a new mum. My parole officer
saying I was using... They just come and took him. Didn't even say, you know, 'I
give you this day to get into rehabilitation or I take your kid.* Izzy Interview 1

The women's sense of powerlessness was evident in the lack of shared decision making around their children who were placed in OOHC For example, Ella, who had five older children in DCJ care was very upset that the foster carer of three of her boys, wanted her children to be christened as Catholic. They had started going to a Catholic school and although she acknowledged that it was the right school for her children, given the limited options in the area where they lived, she did not want them christened as Catholic. Ella's religion is Church of England.

'No, we're Church of England and my mum's gone off, you don't change that
[religion] *you know, you know...I'm not having that'.* Ella Interview 3

Ella was asked about her ability to make decisions about her children, who were in temporary care, however, she was not sure and would have to check with her DCJ worker about this.

Dealing with changing expectations from DCJ was identified as a problematic situation by women who received no notice of these changes and were not allowed to defend themselves. In response, Samara said *'It's so fucked up, man. They promised me'.* She went on to detail her frustration with DCJ, and she felt that no matter what she did it was not going to be good enough. Restoration was possible, but kept getting delayed, and her hopes for restoration with her son was becoming more difficult to imagine as time moved on.

'Cause he was meant to come [home] *this month, and then it was next month'-*
Samara Interview 2

She provided examples of all the courses that she had completed, and services that she had become engaged since going into rehabilitation. Even with these attempts to demonstrate her commitment to parenting she said that DCJ kept moving the goalposts.

'It's so fucked up, man. They promised me. They said, as long as you keep trying
or keep doing what you're supposed to do, then you'll get restoration and now
they have 'taken it off the table altogether' Samara Interview 3

Samara was becoming increasingly frustrated and disparaging towards her DCJ and social care providers. She felt she had no control over anything in her life and was angry when she was interviewed for the third time. She said that DCJ had changed the amount of time she could spend with her son, by half an hour per visit. She was informed that the reason for doing this was that her son could not cope with a longer visit. Samara felt this was very unfair. She mentioned that she was not involved in this decision.

> *Because* [they] *think that the babies can't cope. Zane is the youngest one, and he copes. If he can't cope, fair enough, but they didn't even talk to us mums, or us parents or other carers. They didn't talk to anyone. They just did it, like... I'm pissed. What, because they didn't have fucking time to do it* [supervise the visit]*?...I mean, it gives me the fucking shits.* Samara Interview 3

Theme 3: Constant surveillance and burden of proof

The women described the burden of having to prove to authorities that they were worthy to be a mother. The women wanted to be given the chance by care and social providers to be a parent and appeared to accept that this proof was necessary. At the same time, there was a fine line between having to demonstrate good parenting and being constantly surveyed. Diana, who was in a short-term rehabilitation centre at the time of interview, was informed by DCJ that her baby would be removed if she used any substance. She was really scared about losing custody of her son, and felt she had to demonstrate her ability to mother.

> *'So if I do relapse, the baby will be removed, so I've gotta stay clean...And I've gotta prove to them'... So I've gotta go long-term rehabilitation, and I've gotta change. I've gotta prove to them'* Diana Interview 1

When Diana was interviewed for a second time, and still in the same rehabilitation, she spoke about the difficulties of finding a place to live once she had exited the rehabilitation program. Her wish was to stay with her mother, who was one of her only supports but she was informed that she had to live alone in the community so she could prove to DCJ that she could be a good mother.

> *'Cause they want to see how I am at first when I go outside, in the community. Can I stay drug free out there? Then I can go home, if I can prove that to them'.* Diana Interview 2

A different woman, Cathy who was interviewed at another rehabilitation centre also discussed the need for 'proof'. She had other children removed several years ago when she was in a very violent relationship with her ex-partner. Her children were removed from her care when they were at school one day. Cathy did not get the chance to say goodbye. Sadly, one of these children suffers depression and has made several suicide attempts. He was only nine when his first suicide attempt occurred. Cathy felt that she should have had the chance to prove herself and be provided with the opportunity to parent.

> *Like let me prove myself that, 'yeah I can do this.' And all they had to do before was get me out of the violence instead of take my kids because they didn't just*

Veronica, also discussed the notion of proof and the need to demonstrate her ability to parent.
Veronica, was receiving OAT (buprenorphine) through a pharmacy, and she wanted to have a take
away dose a day or two a week so she did not have to go to the pharmacy every day via public
transport with a newborn infant. She wanted to have some flexibility, and choice. Veronica felt that
first she had to do the right thing, in order to be provided with an opportunity for a takeaway dose.

'Which is fair enough. You do have to prove yourself' Veronica interview 1

When Veronica was interviewed for the second time she had her newborn with her at home.
Veronica discussed how she was instructed to provide urine samples to her doctor. She noted that
this needed to be done so she could show them she was not using. Veronica then described how she
actually hated being monitored. Veronica felt that she could manage her own life, without being
under the spotlight.

*'But yeah, I hate it. I hate it. I have to admit, I hate giving urine samples. I hate
having to go to the chemist. I hate them monitoring me if don't show that I didn't
come yesterday. No, I didn't come yesterday'* Veronica Interview 2

Veronica described herself as a very private person and did not like being monitored. She was
unsure about how long she had to provide urine samples but felt that it could be years. She was
frustrated and upset at the level of surveillance in her life. For example, if she misses picking up her
OAT from the pharmacy, the pharmacy staff call her OAT clinic to let them know that she has missed
a dose.

*They don't call me, they call the drug and alcohol clinic to let them know, and
then the pharmacy can kick me out and say they don't want to dose me anymore
because I'm unreliable or whatever it might be. And you know, it can get
expensive. I mean, you think. Yeah, it only dawned on me a few weeks ago to $40
a week.* Veronica Interview 2

Veronica felt that she was being constantly surveyed and monitored by health and social service
staff for evidence of her mothering. Veronica found this intrusive and confusing. To attest her ability
to be a good mother and prove herself she wanted to have an open and honest relationship with her
care providers. This backfired after she had told them that she had used heroin after the birth of her
baby. Veronica thought that she was doing the right thing by being truthful and informing her care
providers about this occasion but then felt a sense of betrayal when she was reported to DCJ
without her knowledge.

Veronica could not be contacted for her final interview, and she stopped picking up her buprenorphine from the chemist. I am not sure what eventuated for her and her baby, except that there was a lot of concern about this situation from the local substance use in pregnancy team attempted to follow her up.

Samara had supervised visits with her young son and felt that she was being scrutinised constantly during these visits. When I met her for her third interview, she had recently changed lawyers as she felt she was not getting very far with the first one. She appeared desperate and agitated about her situation and found it challenging to navigate her way through the system.

Samara described being closely examined at every step.

> *So I just handed him to her* [another mother], *for a sec, I was pulling at the blanket. And then the DCJ worker comes over and makes this big scene in front of him [her son]. And she goes, 'At no time, should you ever hand your son off to anyone else. You only have two hours. Make the most of it.' And I was like, ' I was trying to put out a blanket.* Samara Interview 3

Veronica was asked whether this process could have been improved and whether it would have been beneficial if services had more transparency about their intentions to report to community services. She replied:

> *I think that would be fair. I just, so then I know what I need to do. Of course stay off drugs and not use. That's a no brainer...but to be told that I should attend counselling every week and just those little things* [to help] *me get off their radar as such.* Veronica Interview 2

The constant surveillance and monitoring experienced by some mothers left one mother feeling paranoid about her interactions with DCJ. For example, when she was given Christmas presents from her DCJ worker for her one year old, she became paranoid that she was being monitored and there were cameras inside the toys.

> *'I was looking for cameras and listening devices, I was being paranoid. And I was thinking are they listening or watching? And my mum said don't be so stupid...you can see they're brand new. You can see the tags'.* Ella Interview 1

Theme 4: The trauma of child removal
The placement of babies and children into OOHC care was understandably distressing for these women. However, the women described differences in the way that this occurred. Some women

were offered support, but others stated there was none or inadequate support. Some women who had children removed into OOHC in the past noted that positively, they were now provided with opportunities to work closely with DCJ to keep their children in their care when it was safe to do so.

When asked why their children were removed into OOHC, the following reasons were provided: substance use (ongoing or a relapse), IPV, late or little engagement with health and social services, and mental health issues. The women were generally experiencing more than one risk factor. For example, Samara and Heather had late engagement with health services during their pregnancies and substance use. In addition, Samara had been experiencing IPV whilst pregnant.

Izzy had relapsed in the community and had minimal support systems in place. However, once she had her son removed into DCJ care, this provided her with a catalyst for change. She described the removal of her son, like she had been 'booted in the guts… no life to live'. She later spent time in a short-term rehabilitation facility. After a short period back in the community she was admitted to a long-term rehabilitation and was now preparing for restoration. She had not had her baby in her care for six months when I met her, but she was having supervised visits with her baby three times a week.

Ella, who had had five children removed when she was experiencing high levels of domestic violence found that the experience has left her holding a lot of hard feelings towards DCJ.

> *'yeah I did and I still do. I hold a lot of hard feelings and then coming into this rehabilitation and all this bullshit'* Ella Interview 1

Ella had a long history with DCJ and with multiple children in OOHC and she had very little trust in the system. She has ongoing anxiety and depression, which she feels is partly due to her children being removed. She also stated that she needed some counselling around this issue. Unfortunately, this counselling was not offered at any point.

Heather, who had two babies removed over two years had quite different experiences. Her first baby was removed when her baby was 12 hours old. However, she spent the first four days with her baby with her second baby, which appreciated, as she was allowed time to bond with him. Although her experience was much better the second time, she still found aspects of it extremely difficult. She disengaged with her DCJ worker in her second pregnancy due to being fearful of having this baby removed, which did occur.

> *'I disengaged with them a bit, I was scared, they had already taken one baby, I didn't want them to take another'* Heather Interview 1

The impact of having little support and her first child removed into OOHC left an indelible mark on Heather and contributed to her disengaging the second time she was pregnant. With her second pregnancy she struggled to motivate herself and get out of bed. She felt depressed.

> *'I was in a state of depression from it* [the fear]. *Wasn't even showering. I remember them saying to me at one stage you need to have a shower. But that was it. That was all they ever said to me...that was it'.* Heather Interview 1

Repercussions of having previous children removed into care was evident for Cathy and how she coped with her most recent pregnancy. She said that she was worried that this child would be removed, like the others were, and so to manage with this fear she used 'ice' pretty much the whole way through her pregnancy.

> *I was just like so afraid to be pregnant again...You know what I mean? Like I was like, 'Oh, no. They're going to take him.' ...and I didn't even think he was going to survive, to be honest. Like, I just thought, 'if I use more it might hurt me if they do take him or if I could lose him in that way.' You know? Like, 'cause the ice takes away feelings, big time.* Cathy Interview 1

At times, the women felt very desperate. Several women expressed feelings of wanting to run, hide and escape reality. One woman identified that she just wanted to take her baby and run. She acknowledged that she had not been engaging with DCJ enough and this was partly because one of her children had been removed in the past and that she was scared that this would happen again.

> *'I didn't wanna ... I didn't wanna have anything to do them. I wanted to run...yeah they'd already taken one of my children away'* Heather Interview 1

One woman reported she ran with her baby straight from the hospital. She had more than five children living in out of home care and was worried they would also remove her newborn, so she fled, with the baby. Nicola had three children before this, who were all living in out of home care and she felt that she has nothing to lose, except to run from the hospital.

> *'And, um, because... I lost him in February, and then...I had a baby in September, and they took him from birth too...Well, I ran from the hospital'.* Nicola Interview 1

The baby was removed and placed in out-of-home care when Nicole was located. Nicola had not received counselling at this point, to deal with her children who were removed. She fell pregnant very soon after this and had another baby, who remained in Nicola's care when we met.

Nicola has ongoing anxiety since her children were removed and taken into care and counselling has never been offered at any point by 'DoCS'. The counselling that she did have, she had to seek it out herself. When asked if she would have found counselling helpful at this point in her life, she replied:

'Yeah, that would have been good too, as I get anxiety from this time… but like everything, all the counselling I got, I sought out myself…It was never offered to me by, with Docs. You know? Like, Docs never offered any help' Nicola Interview 1

One woman was so afraid that her child would be removed into care, like her older child had been, that she hid her pregnancy from everyone until she was eight months pregnant. As a result, neither her partner nor anyone from the rehabilitation centre that she was staying in were aware of her pregnancy. She had hidden this information from everyone as she was scared of what would happen.

'I was scared, I think just of everything…And I look back, and I think, you know, 'That was, that was really, really bad on, on my part.'' Jo Interview 1

Women discussed the difficulties of having children in out of home care and this was in the context of visits, and when they did not go as planned or contact was difficult. Samara spoke about her jealousy, as her son's foster parents got all the 'firsts', such as her baby babbling, smiling, and crawling, while she missed out.

It's just sometimes you know, the, the shit he says and stuff. I'm just like, really? Do you have to tell me that?… like about tummy time and I'm like, don't tell me that shit. You know what I mean? That's my bonding time. Sometimes I think they want to keep him. Samara interview 3

Ella, also expressed frustration with her children being in OOHC. She had five children in OOHC and she commented that she was having issues contacting one of her five boys. The DCJ arrangement was that she can phone him weekly, on a particular day and time but recently she has found it hard to get hold of him.

'We had an agreement, well me and the main carer…. Well the carer said I can ring up every Sunday at three. Yeah. And Sunday I rang and they're not there. I just keep callin' and callin' and they don't pick up'. Ella interview 2.

Ella was worried about her son as he was placed in care, without his siblings. Although, Ella's preference was for her son to be placed with an Aboriginal family, this did not occur.

Theme 5: Sadness and guilt

Mothers expressed sadness and guilt, knowing that some of the choices they have made, and the situations they were in, resulted in negative consequences for their children. The mothers spoke candidly about their experiences of having a newborn with neonatal abstinence disorder (NAS). These women were visibly upset when discussing NAS's impacts on their babies. Several mothers began to cry as they commented on their babies' cries due to NAS. They expanded their comments to include: how hard it was to listen to, and even harder knowing that their actions had lead to their infant's distress

Heather said that it was difficult to hear her baby cry and that her baby is often unsettled. Due to NAS, they had to be cuddled to sleep by the baby's carer (which was not her). She spoke about being upset and disappointed in herself, knowing this was her doing.

> *'I do understand the cuddling him now a bit more-... which I ... It's not something I usually would've done, but I suppose this is my first baby to have, go through withdrawals like this so...I feel really disappointed in myself, no mother likes to see their baby in pain'.* Heather. Interview 1

Samara, whose newborn baby was also placed on morphine for NAS, was scared to see her baby distressed and withdrawing from morphine. She explained that her baby was very unsettled because of the drug withdrawal.

> *'I was scared. Course no one wants to see that, see something that they caused... you know what I mean? And the consequence. You know what I mean? ...Uh, he was really distressed and he was proning'* [laying on his stomach]. Sammy Interview 1

Nicole also expressed guilt and remorse that her daughter had to go through withdrawal because of her choices. She has had five other children and four of these have experienced NAS; though she has never heard a baby cry like her baby did this time. Nicole found this upsetting as the cry of her most recently born baby was the most disturbing and compounded by feeding difficulties:

> *It was horrible, it was really tough to hear and he had a really rough time with the, morphine. Every time he had morphine, he wouldn't feed. He didn't breastfeed or anything, couldn't get him to breastfeed until six weeks old. I'm a decent person, I don't want her to go through withdrawals because of my choices in life* Nicola Interview 1

Theme 6: Catch 22- being set up to fail

The women described being placed in situations that hindered their ability to stay drug-free and safe and return home with their babies. This included being placed in social housing where there was a high prevalence of drug use, having problems accessing IPV support and counselling, and issues around being able to parent effectively.

Izzy was living in a Department of Housing unit with her young son who was six months old. The building was a large inner-city tower block with multiple social housing blocks all within very close vicinity. The towers are well known to house and be frequented by people with a history of SUDs and people with a history of incarceration and other social and economic issues.

Initially, Izzy received support through her DCJ worker, however, her case had been closed and DCJ assessed her to be doing well. Izzy said that she became lonely and started associating with the 'wrong crowd' and tempted to use drugs enabling her to be a part of a group. She said she did not know how to say 'no' when offered drugs. She said that there were drugs everywhere.

> *'Too much … Too much drugs…*[you can] *get them anywhere'* Izzy Interview 1

Being exposed to substance use and its impact was also explained by Faith. She was in a rehabilitation clinic with her baby and there were drugs everywhere in the clinic; this temptation was instrumental in her demise. She said she developed another habit while staying in the rehabilitation setting.

> *It wasn't the same manager, and all the girls that were here before, they were all using, so there was drugs here, the whole time I was here…And it was so hectic, and I kept telling DOCS, and I'm telling them to please get me out of here. I don't want to be here, there's drugs everywhere, and you know? I'm trying to tell them, and they didn't believe me.* Faith Interview 1

One woman mentioned that she didn't feel comfortable with the plan that DCJ had made for her when she was discharged from the rehabilitation clinic back into the community. Diana wanted to go into long-term rehabilitation and then home with her mother, who she said could provide some stability and support for her and her newborn infant. However, DCJ preferred that she live in independent housing in the community so they could assess her parenting ability. Again, she felt she was being set up to fail.

> *Well, you know, I'm trying to go to* [long term rehab] *and I want to be able to go back home so it's kind of … that part is kind of not supportive* [from DCJ], *where they would like me to rent a property and live in the community…you know, having a baby and to have no support and to not have money, financially. They're just setting me up to fail.* Diana Interview 2

When she was interviewed, Natalie was five months pregnant, was homeless, using CMA, and had two other children who had been previously taken into OOHC. She spoke about one time after she had given birth with her now two year old daughter when she was in hospital and wanting to feed her baby. However, she felt that whatever she had done was not good enough, and she was being constantly scrutinised every step of the way. One time, she had wanted to feed her baby, but was told she needed to rest, and then when she did, she was told she was ignoring her baby.

> *With my daughter they* [hospital staff] *were telling me when she was hungry, but I know, when she's hungry.. And I was like, Okay. I'll put a bottle on and she said, no, no, no, no, no, no, no problem, you sit down you've got your hands full... I'll do it, and them she said, I ignored her* [the baby], *who was due to be fed. They said she was hungry and crying and I totally completely ignored her.* Natalie Interview 1

Finally, Ash described how she had tried to get onto methadone when she was pregnant but had to go on a waiting list, so she just kept using

> *'Like the reason why I kept using is because I, I was trying to get on the methadone treatment- And then they kept saying, 'No, you've got to go on a waiting list...And I'm like, 'Well, I can't wait, so I've got to use again and again, and again-'* Ash Interview 1

The women discussed how difficult it was for men to access IPV support services, as perpetrators of violence, which meant that even though they were attending DV programs, this did not make any difference as their partners where not accessing services. In addition, two women discussed that they wanted to keep the family unit together and felt let down by the system and felt that there was not enough support for men. These two women acknowledged that they needed to be apart from their partners as the risk of IPV was high, but they still loved them, so this was a difficult trade-off.

Ash spoke about the times that her partner was violent towards her was when he had been using ice. He would experience a psychosis, which would often end in an assault. She wanted him to access treatment and support, but he was not doing so, this meant she could not stay with him.

> *'I think he went somewhere, and he spoke to someone, a counsellor and stuff like that but he never got back in touch with them'* Ash Interview 3

This issue was further compounded by the fact that Ash still loved her partner and wanted him to be part of her life. The following comment demonstrates this:

Yeah, it's not as simple as …[he] has to be supported…because a lot of times you're like…I *still love* him *and it's, yeah, it's very hard to just walk away…um … You know, I keep giving him chances. It goes like, I can see the two different people like who he used to be and how he is now.* Ash Interview 3

Izzy noted that as she had been seeking assistance and support around her drug use and her IPV, her partner needed to step up to the plate if he wanted any chance of seeing their son.

It's been about three weeks now, because every time he'd ring up, I'd hang up, and well, I'd tell him that I don't want, don't want to talk to him, because I told him, 'I feel like you kno-, know what you need to do if you want to be a part of your son's life. Like I've got to do it, so if you want to be a father, you've got to do it too, you know? Izzy Interview 1

The issues of dealing with IPV within the already complex lives of these women is evident from the quote from Natalie. She was interviewed while in a short-term rehabilitation setting. Unfortunately, Natalie left the rehabilitation clinic before the end of the program and did not regain custody of her young baby. Instead, she felt that she was being punished because of the IPV, which she could not stop; and the outcome was that she did not gain custody of her child.

'He lost his job. He had carpal tunnel, he started hitting me, he was using drugs, he wasn't paying rent, then they crucified me for domestic violence and no one helped me' Natalie Interview 1

The complexities of these situations were acknowledged by one woman who described the difficulties of extricating yourself from a situation when you still love that person.

Theme 7: Desire for a normal life

Despite the hardships, stressors and instabilities present in these women's lives, many continued to have hope for the future. They valued the positive interactions they had with health and social care providers and wanted to be given a chance to be a mother and live a normal life, as well as appreciating the moments they spent with their newborns, even if it was a short period.

Faith spoke highly of her DCJ worker. She referred to her DCJ worker as a 'miracle worker' and went 'above and beyond' to help her gain a sense of normality. Faith was homeless, living on the streets and was experiencing IPV. She was almost full-term when she met her DCJ worker in regional NSW. Faith was very grateful for the support and opportunity she provided to be a mother to her newborn infant.

> *This woman is like a miracle worker...Yeah, this is what she done for me. She*
> *picked me up and she took me down to the clinic, and she got then to open the*
> *doors up, and she phoned a prescribing doctor to meet us there...Yeah, and yeah,*
> *she's just done so much for me.* Faith Interview 1

Cathy also benefited from a positive relationship with her DCJ worker as she praised her initial worker as someone who gave her a second chance. Unfortunately, she had to change workers.

> *'Um, well I had the best DCJ worker that I've ever had. For so long... and he like*
> *but now he's just passed me over to someone else'.* Cathy Interview 1

When asked what was so important about their relationship? She said, 'well he had given me that second chance'.

Heather spoke about how she was grateful to be provided with the opportunity to spend some bonding time with her newborn before her baby was removed into DCJ care. This time provided her with a snapshot of being a Mum. With her most recent pregnancy, she was allowed to be by her baby's bedside as much as she wanted, which compared to her last pregnancy was a very different experience when her baby was removed when they were 12 hours old.

> *'Yeah, and I was able to just have my little bonding time with him. We build a nice*
> *strong bond. Yeah'* Heather Interview 1

Heather spent four days with her baby before he was removed into care. Even though she said this was a different outcome than what she had expected, and she was unprepared, the removal happened in a supportive way, and there was a social worker that worked closely with her and helped her get into a rehabilitation as soon as she was discharged from hospital.

Unfortunately, when I met Heather several months after our interview, she had left rehabilitation and relapsed and had gone back to her partner who was using drugs heavily at the time. At our interview, when she was in rehabilitation she was worried about her partner, and that he was not getting the help that he needed for his substance use.

When Heather was asked what support she thought was needed at the time, she responded that she wanted to be able to have a family home.

> *'I want to have a family home, that's what I want in the end... if there were*
> *services ... we could be supported as a family unit, then that would be perfect'.*
> Heather Interview 1

Ash had a similar experience, as she felt she had to choose between her and her partner. Her partner had a history of violence towards her and mental health issues, and he was using crystal methamphetamine at times. Ash was aware that in order to keep herself and her children safe, she needed to distance herself from him. The dilemma was that they had been together on and off for many years and she still loved him. She wished that he could get the help that he needed but said that he found it difficult to access the right support at the right time. Ash identified that keeping her partner at a distance was difficult. The following comment demonstrates this.

> *I actually rang them* [the DCJ worker] *and I said, look can you make him do the mental health stuff…yeah because I think for a lot of women they have to choose between their husband and their family, but a lot of people want both you know. And it's not that they don't want their kids, they just don't know how to push the husband away, and in not doing that they end up losing their children.* Ash interview 3

Some of the women commented on the structure and routine such as those provided to them in rehabilitation, which demonstrated the yearning for normalcy. For example, two women discussed the worth of having structure in their day, and how this was beneficial for them, and their babies. Jo stated that she and her son were enjoying rehabilitation, the routine, and that her son is now doing well.

> *He is settling in, he is much more settled now…you know, he'll be up, we- we'll both be up and out about 6:00, and, um, yeah, have breakfast and- then go down to childcare, while we have our group… then back to childcare again while we have our afternoon group.* Jo Interview 1

Diana similarly mentioned that she found value in the routine, and that because of this she felt much healthier

> *'We get three meals. And I sleep every night the same time, I get up at the same time. So everything is routine. So I can feel my body is so much healthier'.* Diana Interview 1

Chapter summary

Despite all the challenges these women and their children face, hope and self-belief was a prominent feature. Women were asked: what their hopes for the future were, and predominantly these women wanted a 'normal life'. They wanted the opportunity to parent their children, live in the community and be part of a family unit. These following comments reflect the sentiment of these women and how they remained positive in such challenging times.

'I truly believe in myself, especially having a baby, I don't want it to, as much as I've got extra stress and stuff, I don't feel like I would even want to go and use'. Veronica interview 2

Unfortunately for these women, their hopes to parent their children were limited or cut off completely by systems that they identified as setting them up to fail. This was due to a lack of suitable housing, appropriate support, and involvement in violent relationships that left them scared and traumatised. In addition, some women's substance use was so chaotic that it would have been unsafe for children to remain in their care. The following two chapters describe the findings from the views on women's experiences from health and social care providers, and DCJ workers.

CHAPTER EIGHT: PHASE THREE QUALITATIVE FINDINGS OF HEALTH CARE WORKERS

Thirteen health care workers took time out of their busy workday to be interviewed for this study. Five nurses, two midwives, one addiction medicine specialist, one neonatologist, two social workers, a social work student and a rehabilitation manager provided important insights into the needs of pregnant women and new mothers with a history of IDU. Of the 13 workers, 12 were very experienced in their field. The doctors were senior consultants, the midwives had been working for over 15 years each and the five nurses had a minimum of ten years of nursing experience. The two social workers had been working for five years each. Finally, the rehabilitation manager worked professionally for over 20 years, having worked with marginalised and vulnerable women for over a decade.

The health care workers that participated in the interviews were passionate and dedicated professionals who advocated for positive outcomes for this group of women, and their children when they were involved in their care. The interviews suggest that they were working in a very niche area of health care that was often stigmatised, and underfunded. In addition, they had to manage the complex care needs of clients who often presented with SUDs, mental health disorders including underlying trauma and medical issues such as hepatitis C.

Eight themes that emerged from the analysis of the interview data from the health care workers. These themes were: Stigma and its consequence, with the sub-themes of health care stigma and consequences of stigma. Other themes were competing priorities, access to care, child removal, falling through the cracks, power, violence and mother's determination.

Theme 1: Stigma and its consequences

Stigma was a prominent feature that was discussed by nearly all the health and social care providers. They were stigmatised because of the nature of their work and because of who they provide care to. The health care workers commented on the impact that stigma has on their clients. One doctor voiced concern that the high levels of stigma in the workforce lead to high staff attrition rates, which can affect client outcomes. He said that some workers go into the profession because they are altruistic. Unfortunately, workers are then stigmatised and become disillusioned due to people not always getting better, or they realise they share different values with their clients that cannot be reconciled, so they leave. The doctor felt that stigma was the main driver behind the ongoing staffing issues in the sector.

'I think the stigma is probably the single biggest factor driving people out of this area'
Patrick, Addiction medicine specialist

Beside the notion of stigma affecting the workforce, Patrick discussed the ongoing presence of stigma in mainstream hospital settings, and maternity services and how this effects patients. Even though the program for mothers with SUDs had been there for many years, this stigma is present.

> *'The interactions with the obstetrics and maternity services are very difficult for them [the women] And they remain highly stigmatised...this hospital's had a drugs and pregnancy service for 25 or 30 years... and they still have major conflicts'* Patrick, Addiction medicine specialist

Additionally, another doctor echoed Patrick's comments regarding stigma. She felt that stigma could be related to high burn-out, and consequently this could mean that care could be fragmented.

> *'Yeah, there's a high burn-out...And I think there needs to be a lot more talking between the area health services... there is a lot of silo's, unfortunately'* Jane, Neonatologist

The s health care workers were asked: what is one of the biggest challenges that pregnant women and mothers with SUD face? For one, health care workers she said it was fear, stigma, and discrimination. Natalie, a midwife and a nurse, has worked in this area of health for over ten years supporting many pregnant women with SUDS. Natalie provided many examples of when her clients have had negative experiences within health care settings because of stigma. She said that her clients have been labelled injecting drug uses when they have not been, and they have been assumed to have hepatitis C when it had been a past infection. She spoke of her frustrations when reading referral forms for pregnant women that state the women is a drug user, a sex worker, and they have hepatitis C. At the end of the referral, it would then mention they're pregnant. This frustrated Natalie as the pregnancy was the main issue, and she felt that mainstream health professionals made many assumptions.

> *I've read discharge summaries from our clients if they've gone to emergency [and] it's like homeless and sex working and you read Hep C positive. Oh and then they're pregnant. And then, you know, I have to ring those clinicians and go, actually they're not hep c positive. If you asked them the question or done the right test, you'd know. Natalie, midwife and registered nurse*

Natalie described a situation she experienced with a pregnant woman who went to the hospital for an issue completely unrelated to her pregnancy. Here she felt judged as she divulged that she was on a methadone program. The client stated that she felt that everyone was looking at her because she was pregnant and on methadone. The provider's response was confusing as she thought that being on methadone was the right thing to do.

> *'It was such a big step for her to even engage in that process to begin with. And it kind of set her back in her perception of the fact that she was actually doing something good for herself and her baby by being on the program* [methadone]'. Natalie, midwife and registered nurse

Two other midwives employed in a tertiary setting discussed in detail the stigma that hospital staff had towards this group of mothers and how they were made to feel guilty. One midwife said that the mothers 'started off on the back foot', and were judged by hospital staff, especially if they had a baby in the special care nursery due to NAS. The second midwife regularly asked her clients about their experiences of being on the antenatal ward, the mothers mostly said that they have had a negative experience as they felt that others were talking about them.

> *'They're wondering what everybody is thinking about you and, and you know, there will be whispers'.* Clare, clinical midwife consultant

The issue with staff discrimination against this group of women can lead to women not receiving the care they need as they are judged for their actions. Annie, who is one of the midwives mentioned above and whose primary role is to support pregnant women and new mothers with SUDs describes the following:

> *The main stigma, will come from staff. I've had numerous conversations with the NUMS* [nursing unit managers] *about how staff will approach our clients. I don't know how you would call it. They're a bit standoffish. Oh, they've already got an opinion on the clients, and they've already made a judgment before they actually go in and talk to them. Annie, clinical midwife consultant*

> *'And when* [asked], *how have you been treated, do you feel that you've been treated well? Most of them say no'.* Annie, clinical midwife consultant

Stigma was experienced by both health and social care workers. The consequences of stigma included: inadequate funding, high staff turnover, poor access to contraception services and limited support for breastfeeding.

Leanne, a women's rehabilitation centre manager, felt that due to the nature of the work provided at her service, there is limited opportunity to apply for extra funding as people are less inclined to fund services for people with SUDs. Leanne felt that if she worked in a service that provided care for less controversial issues such as cancer care, there would be more funding opportunities.

I can go for funding [and] *you say, cancer, everybody's heart goes out... Drug and alcohol, 'Oh she does it to herself' you know? Nobody wants to. So you know, the, the angle I take nowadays in funding is always talking about, these children didn't want to be the children of alcoholics or substance using parents.* Leanne, rehabilitation manager

One social worker felt the stigma associated with SUD meant that women sometimes found it hard to access contraception. For example, she said that one woman expressed fear of being asked too many questions about her current situation and that in the course of the consult it may become apparent she was using drugs. This stigma for women is the general avoidance of health care environments altogether. The following comment demonstrates this situation:

'I just had a, a session with a client who hasn't had any contraception, and she has said that if I went to my doctor, he would know I was using'. Nikki, Social worker

Unfortunately, the consequences of stigma for this group of women also mean mothers do not feel equipped or confident to breastfeed. Two midwives spoke about how hard it was for this group of women to breastfeed, primarily due to staff's stigma and judgemental attitudes who labelled them 'drug users'.

'I mean, you'll get the underlying judgment that this mum's done it. So you don't deserve to have this baby. Look at these poor parents who gone through IVF, look at this, How dare they [breastfeed]'. Clare clinical midwife consultant

One of the midwives, also a lactation consultant spoke about the clear benefits of breastfeeding in this cohort of women. Two major benefits for the women were: bonding between the mother and infant and increasing self-esteem for the mother that she could do something positive as a mother, despite everything else that was happening in her life. She also mentioned that research has found that breastfeeding can be a mitigating factor for child abuse.

As a lactation consultant, she may sometimes get called in to help a mother discontinue breastfeeding as the child is going into OOHC. She said even if the mother would like to continue breastfeeding, DCJ puts up brick walls and makes it difficult to do so, despite the known positive benefits for both mother and baby.

They're removing their child, severing that sort of tie, they're putting a sort of shield around the baby. So they've protected the baby, but really have no understanding of the importance of the attachment to the mother, from the child's point of view. Clare, clinical midwife consultant

Theme 2: Competing priorities in women's lives

Heath and social care providers discussed that it was hard to address multiple issues present for women when there was just so much to do. One of the nurses and a midwife identified the limited resources to cope with these competing priorities and complex issues. For example, women may be struggling with breastfeeding, have to attend meetings with DCJ, do a UDS, and pick up methadone daily. In addition, they may be at risk or experiencing IPV, while at the same time having sex and not on contraception and worrying about falling pregnant. The accumulation of these competing priorities and complex issues can mean that the women are overburdened. The women are then likely to make choices, that may make their lives easier but this may not always be the best for them or their baby.

One midwife quoted the following:

> It's really hard because these women have got bigger hurdles to jump and they're less equipped to be able to do it. Maybe they have to pick up their methadone, or meet deadlines. It's hard when you got a baby that just might feed at any time. So [mothers think] if I can give them a bottle and then I know they're going to sleep this long and settle, I've got this much gap, you know, I've got this many hours and maybe, or the baby will sleep longer at night. Clare, clinical midwife consultant

Health care workers were asked to explain how they thought women perceived contraception. Sally, a nurse, felt that the women just had so much going on in their lives, and that accessing contraception was far from their minds. While some women may want to have a baby even if the outcome may not be optimal. The following comment demonstrates this.

> Maybe they're having a baby and they really want to make a family or they want to tie somebody to them. I don't often say it, but why would you do, you know you've already got two kids, and hold on, shit I'm having sex and I can get pregnant. They're pushed to the brink and they still don't [access contraception]...it's that living moment to moment. Sally, clinical nurse consultant

Patrick, the addiction medicine specialist, also mentioned the issue of priorities and contraception. He felt that this was way down the bottom of the women's list this was compounded by general chaos that existed in these women's lives resulting in contraception not being on their radar.

> 'But, but the women, women were not generally interested because of their, I think more than anything, um, they, they had multiple completing-competing priorities, a lot of chaos in their lives and incredible ambivalence towards everything'. Patrick, Addiction medicine specialist

Theme 3: Access to care

Several health care workers discussed the high levels of unresolved mental health issues present in this group of women, and how it is difficult to disentangle from the underlying levels of trauma. For example, one of the interviewed midwives finds that the state wide NSW Health Domestic Violence screening tool is not of much use, and that women lie anyway. She also suspects that many of the women have undiagnosed mental health conditions.

> *'I actually think most of them lie. Because they've all got mental health issues also linked to the DV are mental health issues, but like which one came first?... they all have undiagnosed depression and mild anxiety'* Annie clinical midwife consultant

Annie's suggested that meaningful interactions with women over time, and rapport building, provides a better sense of where the woman was in regard to her mental health.

According to the health care worker interviews, access to good and consistent mental health care can be difficult. Two health care workers working in a rehabilitation setting discussed the challenges they have when they want to obtain a mental health assessment for their clients. The rehabilitation centre manager said that she has been working for 18 months to get an effective system in place, which consists of a thorough psychiatric review. She has found support for acute care issues, as there is a local acute care team available, but for the mothers who need assessment for chronic mental health care it has been a difficult road to navigate.

> *'So that's a that's a very very big gap, and we're trying to find, we're trying to bridge that gap because right now I'm talking to them saying, "I don't want just a medication review, I want a psychiatric review".* Leanne, rehabilitation manager

One of the social workers spoke about how hard it was to get services to focus on trauma care, and instead some clinicians will focus on the drug and alcohol issues as a separate issue to the mental health issue. This can mean that a woman will have to have two separate assessments, one for the drug and alcohol issue and then a mental health assessment, instead of focusing on trauma informed care, being the trauma as the underlying issue.

> *Some clinicians think drug and alcohol and mental health are quite separate. You know, they need to have a separate assessment and they ... Drug and alcohol needs to see them and treat that box and then mental health needs to see them and treat them', rather than it being trauma focused.* Kristina, social worker

Similarly, Natalie, a nurse and midwife also identified the challenges these women experienced accessing mental health assessments. Natalie said that health care workers make assumptions about a person's history, they do not always take a thorough mental health history and therefore blame the drug use, on the mental health disorder or the mental health disorder on the drug use which becomes a 'chicken and egg' scenario.

> *There's a perception of these women in hospital, of mental illness, or if they're using methamphetamines, that they have psychosis from drug use. Not that anyone looked at their past mental health history and realised that they've got mental health diagnosis* [that's] *exacerbated by methamphetamine use.* Natalie, midwife, registered nurse

Waiting lists for treatment were mentioned as an access issue where health care workers spoke about long waiting lists for access to SUD treatment programs. Lists were particularly long at some times a year, such as Christmas when some treatment centres closed or limited their client intake.

> *'For example, with December, you are like … screwed- lots of the rehabs close their wait list and so, if you have someone who's say, unbooked, it is very hard to get them in'* Kristina, social worker

In addition, there is not a one size fits all treatment model and often women need to take whatever is available to them. Whether they feel this treatment service is best for them is irrelevant, especially if the women are being told they must enter the rehabilitation program or have their baby removed.

> *'So the woman has to take whatever's around-whether it's going to suit her needs or not...and you almost know by accepting that, you probably really risking them being exited* [asked to leave] *but- they're just kind of desperate and if it means having your baby removed or going to this rehab- you just have to take the latter'* Kristina, social worker

Theme 4: Child removal and trauma

Health and social care providers discussed situations where women had children removed from their care and how this could make or break women. One social worker noted that removing a child into OOHC provided some women with an opportunity to engage with services, and make contact with their baby, or child, but some mothers go 'underground'. Kristina said that often a woman will self-discharge from the hospital as soon as the baby is removed into OOHC, and re-engagement and follow up is difficult. Kristina stated the following:

> *'Most of the time, women discharge themselves really quickly, after an assumption of care and they stop breastfeeding straight away'.* Kristina, social worker

Kristina stated that some health care workers she had worked with believe that a baby should not get 'too attached' to their mother if removal is inevitable. However, Kristina did not think this should be the case, and the women she spoke to about a pending removal want to stay with their baby for as long as possible. Some women even want to continue breastfeeding post removal. If the hospital supports this, it can keep a woman on the wards just that little longer, and they feel connected to their baby, even when they cannot be there to parent.

> 'It [breastfeeding] *gave them a sense of purpose, in the sense of it is a good motivation to stay clean because they knew that they had to sort of stay ... and it gave them a sense that they, they couldn't care for their baby full time but they could do this'* Kristina, social worker

Removing a child into OOHC was understandably a very distressing time for women. In addition, health care workers discussed how they also found it hard, especially if the mother was ill-prepared or struggling to accept the situation. One midwife spoke about a time when she was involved in a child removal situation that was particularly difficult for all concerned, especially the mother. The mother would not let go of her baby when the time came for the baby to be removed into care. She recalls this as a very traumatic moment.

> '*But we're all, you know, in tears and it was just the most horrific thing I've ever done. Oh my God. You know, and I've seen everything. Actually she wouldn't hand it over to anyone else, so it was terrible. Oh, still. She, they're working towards restoration. There is hope'.* Annie, clinical midwife consultant

A social worker and nurse who both work in a rehabilitation centre were asked to comment on their experiences working with women who have had children removed into care. Nic, the social worker stated that if there is a history of past child removal, then 'they're re-traumatised all over again'. The nurse said she was not aware if women were offered counselling or not at this moment however, it would not be of much use as the women are in shock at that point.

> '*It's too soon, they don't even know what's happening at the point'.* Frankie, clinical nurse specialist

Natalie, a midwife spoke about the trauma of child removal and linked it to a possible reason why women are ambivalent about the use of contraception.

> '*There's always that one baby. They might let me take home...if I get pregnant again and I can sort my shit out and maybe I'll get to go home with this baby? eventually they'll let me take this baby home'.* Natalie, midwife, registered nurse

Theme 5: Falling through the gaps

This theme describes the barriers women face receiving ongoing, consistent and appropriate care that meets their needs. Two nurses working in substance use and pregnancy spoke about their frustrations with the gaps in the system for this group of women. Their team is multidisciplinary and provides care and support to these women during their pregnancy and up until the baby is 18 months old. After this time, there is a question about who supports these women and their children. The nurses noted that this this is a critical time for mother and her child, and it was concerning that no-one was necessarily actively following-up the these women and their babies.

> *'You've got this big gap. So my frustration and challenge is what should go in that gap. That's a talk that's evolving. But it is quite challenging because it's like whose client are they? Are they D&As* [drug and alcohol]?- *they may not be using anymore? I find that really frustrating'* Sally, clinical nurse consultant

The solution provided was that the mother and child should be assertively followed up, until the child begins school.

> *If we'd have stayed involved for five years, the child potentially might not be removed. They might not relapse. It just doesn't make sense. It's more cost effective to have the team that engage with them'* Sally, clinical nurse consultant

Another perinatal health worker Charlie also discussed gaps in services. She was concerned that issues arose when a mother needed to transition from a hospital setting caring for low-risk pregnant women to a different hospital setting that cares for high-risk pregnant women. This may occur if the woman's needs become more complex. Charlie spoke about the difficulties of transferring care for women with SUDs, as they can take time to develop trust and rapport with health care workers. Her experience was that women can fall through the cracks and may disengage from care altogether. Charlie's preference was to continue to follow these women up, even if they moved to a setting that could better meet their needs.

> *'So we will just hand them over to* [another setting] *because we are not allowed to continue the care. So, we are going to lose them, they will have some gap in engagement, where here, they already trust us'* Charlie social worker

This gap in continuation of care was discussed by a midwife who felt that some women completely fall off the service's radar once they go home with their baby. At times, this can be detrimental to the well-being and development of the child, especially for those women that are not engaged in early childhood and family services.

Annie noted that a new case model system was commencing, which meant that women and their children would be proactively followed up for two years postnatally, by child and family health. It was not clear if they would be followed up after these two years, but she felt that it was a good start.

'Two years. Up to two years. So the whole thing start to finish. So when the child hits two, I don't know where they'll go...it's more to keep an eye on them. Cause at the moment, if you don't want [to go to] *child family health, you don't need to, nobody follows them up'* Annie, clinical midwife consultant

Several barriers were known to impact follow up care for women who had children removed into OOHC. The health care workers identified these barriers to included limited or inadequate referral pathways, and women being lost to follow up due to transience or disconnected mobile phones.

Kristina, a perinatal social worker, found it frustrating that she could not follow up clients whose children had been removed into OOHC once they were discharged from hospital. This was primarily because this was not part of her remit, which set women up to fail. Clients were mostly referred to another service for follow up after discharge. Still, Kristina found that women were not amenable to meeting another person at this point, or they were uncontactable. Instead, women ended up in crisis, and came back to the hospital seeking care. Kristina lamented over this situation and wished she could provide continuing care.

'Lots of my clients would come back to see me in a crisis. But I wasn't able to [see them]- *Like, I mean, we probably bent the rules a bit, in terms of being flexible. But I wasn't able to provide any follow up'* Kristina, social worker

In addition, play groups that cater for women and their children with histories of a SUD were noted to be useful by one midwife. Women felt more comfortable around other women in similar situations, and less judged. Unfortunately, there are very few of these specialist play groups.

The availability of resources and effective collaboration between health professionals was an issue brought to the attention of one medical officer. He stated that because the clients had such complex needs, more intense resourcing was required. In addition, all health workers, who worked with women with SUDs, need to work collaboratively, which sometimes was not the case. He identified that often women required coordinated care from multiple health care professionals simultaneously including obstetrics, neonatology, medical, nursing, allied health, social workers, community, psychiatry, and drug and alcohol services. To further complicate this care, the often- underlying pathology such as hepatitis C needs addressing.

When asked how effective these different services were at collaborating, he replied: 'well they don't'. He felt that part of the problem was that the whole area is stigmatised and attracts less resources. Even if the resources are available, stigma is still an issue. The following comment demonstrates this:

> *By the time that a woman may come in for an appointment, they may have already encountered several levels of stigma along the way- this may be from the bus on the way in, or the receptionist at a clinic, and so you spend the first 15 minutes of the appointment calming the person down'.* Patrick, addiction medicine specialist

Differing organisational philosophies of different rehabilitation programs meant that women would receive varying degrees of health advice. For example, one rehabilitation program was 100% abstinence based. As a result, women could be discharged for smoking on site, and sugar was rationed. Because the service was abstinence-based, this also meant that harm reduction messages were not discussed.

> *'We're abstinent based, but then you know, we're not saying* [no] *harm minimum, but we don't talk about it because it's, ours is only abstinent based'* Leanne, rehabilitation manager

Theme 6: Power

Power over women was pervasive in health care settings. Midwives discussed power imbalances between a new mother and her baby. One midwife, Clare stated that ward staff often act like the baby is theirs and have ownership over the baby as the women are in 'their' ward. It was noted that this could be intimidating for any new mother, especially for mothers with SUDs who are often disempowered from the start. Clare said that mothers with SUDs could feel very intimidated by this power imbalance, as is demonstrated by the following comment:

> *'I don't know what I'm allowed to do...I've got to be really nice to you because you're between you and my baby and if I'm not nice to you, you might not be nice to my baby. So I'm going to be really passive and subservient and submissive'* Clare, clinical midwife consultant

There were powers that DCJ workers could institute that other health care workers could not concerning child protection outcomes. For instance, one health worker found it very frustrating that at times she did not understand the decisions made by DCJ, and felt that, no matter what a woman did, it was just not good enough because DCJ kept changing the goals posts. It was mentioned that this may be because they are from differing philosophies – DCJ viewed their work through a child lens, whereas they were more involved in the direct care of the mother.

> *We say, and because the God in child protection terms, we have no leeway. We have no leverage. We can't do anything'… 'But it's, it's very annoying when we're working with the families, getting them to a point and we think they're good… And then they* [DCJ] *turn around and saying, no, we want more from you. But they never said this in the beginning. They seem to change the goal posts.* Annie, clinical midwife consultant

The two midwives felt that their experience and knowledge of the situation were undermined. They worked very closely with the women they provided care for and felt that even through the perinatal family conferencing, DCJ still had the final say. In a different incident, the health care workers recommended that DCJ not send a baby home with their mother, as they did not feel safe to do so. However, DCJ had the final say and the baby went home. Tragically, the baby had a fractured skull not soon after returning home.

> 'So everybody at the hospital was saying don't send the baby home. Yeah. But DCJ got the final say' Annie, clinical midwife consultant

Despite the frustrations that health and social care providers had with DCJ, interactions with DCJ workers were generally positive, even if there were differing opinions on how things should be managed. Health care workers felt that the best way to approach the relationship between their clients and DCJ workers was to support the work that DCJ do. This willingness to work together was demonstrated by the following comments by two health care workers.

> '*Yeah, it's all variable* [the relationship]… *Yeah… We try and build solid connections with them though*' Frankie, clinical nurse specialist

> '*I always try and frame it to the women that they are here to help and they are doing a job and looking after you and looking after your baby. And we might not always agree with what they say, but they have a purpose and that purpose can be really helpful*' Natalie, midwife, registered nurse

Health care workers also acknowledged that the relationship between DCJ workers and their clients can be strained. This strained relationship is even more so when the women have had children removed by DCJ. This means that it can be challenging to convince women that they need to work closely and collaborate with DCJ.

> ' the relationship is strained, so coming in on a strained relationship is always difficult. Um, but I'd say that, you know, we work really hard with them' Natalie, midwife, registered nurse.

Theme 7: Violence

Many health care workers mentioned IPV as one of the greatest challenges facing women with SUDs. It was also a significant challenge for health care workers, to manage. Some women did not want to address the issue, and there seemed to be a level of acceptance of violence in their lives. Additionally, some women did not recognise that what they were experiencing could be classified as IPV, or they had lost faith in the system to protect them from the effects of IPV.

Health care workers discussed the multiple services and legal processes available to mitigate the effects of IPV such as Safety Action Management, counselling, perinatal family conferencing, apprehended violence orders (AVOs) and programs through DCJ such as Staying Home Leaving Violence. Of significance was that health care workers reported that women often find these programs futile.

> '99% of them won't accept any help [with IPV]'. Annie, clinical midwife consultant

> 'It is another challenge because we have had women who come here, who are in fear of their lives but don't wanna take action by getting an AVO'. Lorraine, social worker

The role of AVOs seemed to be a particularly contentious issue, where women have lost faith in the system due to systems failures.

> 'Sometimes, but more than often the women don't that AVO in place because well...they see it as being useless because they [the male partner] always breach it and they only go back to jail for a week or two...challenging' Jill, clinical nurse consultant

Jill, a perinatal clinical nurse consultant, said that IPV is rife in the community of women that she provides care for and IPV creates a complicated situation for all concerned. Jill said that she makes it very clear that women who are experiencing IPV, are informed that they need to do something about it if they want to keep their baby in their care, and for their safety.

'We make it really clear this is so dangerous. You can't stay with him If you're going to have your baby at home, then that's what's going to happen. Yeah. So get away from, get to a refuge, get to rehab, do stop, you know what I mean? Just basically get out of it'. Jill, clinical nurse consultant

Theme 8: Mothers' Determination

Despite the complex challenges for mothers with SUD, some women exhibited enormous strength and resilience. These women were determined to continue to mother, even in the physical absence of their babies. This is evident in how the women wanted to continue breastfeeding even when the children have been removed from their care. With support and encouragement from care providers, it was noted that there were multiple benefits by encouraging women to breastfeed, even in the absence of their children. Firstly, it would keep the women on the ward for longer which means that more medical and social needs could be addressed post-partum, and secondly, women felt that they had a sense of purpose and could still care for their child even when they weren't there.

The feedback that we got from women, was that it, it gave them a sense of purpose, in the sense of like uh, one, it was like a good motivation to stay clean because they knew that they had to sort of stay ... It gave them a sense that they, they couldn't care for their baby full time but they could do this thing. Kristina, perinatal social worker

Two workers discussed the positive outcomes that can be achieved if the mother is determined to work with service providers. Kristine spoke about a woman she had worked with who had previously had five children removed into OOHC. She said her client was determined to do things differently and wanted to enact positive change.

'I worked with families that might have had like five children removed from their care. And seeing how they can make kind of changes, in such a small period of time, actually, it is amazing to witness.' Kristina, social worker

Leanne mentioned similar situations where mothers, if they collaborate with services and are driven to change, positive outcomes can follow.

'...and they have hope for the future...but still there's hope, you know? There's something in them that makes them say, 'I wanna do it,' and they come here. And to see the process, that change, you know?' Leanne, rehabilitation centre manager

Natalie elaborated further the positive outcomes when women are empowered. Natalie mentioned that women who participate in the perinatal family conferencing and are engaged in the process and want to do well can keep their babies post birth. For example, Natalie provided support to a woman engaged in her antenatal care, commencing a methadone program for her heroin use, and participating in perinatal family conferencing meetings. As a result, she went home straight from the hospital at day five with her newborn, who was weaning off morphine for NAS. Natalie noted it was important to focus on the strengths that women displayed and remind the women of their achievements along the way.

> *'That can be a really empowering process for women as well and you can just keep going back to look at the strengths. There are so many things that they have achieved and they need to keep remembering that.'* Natalie nurse and midwife

The baby that Natalie was referring to in the above scenario tragically died of sudden infant death syndrome some weeks post-discharge. The mother was very distressed by this outcome and disengaged from many services. She started smoking large quantities of marijuana and was at risk of losing her older children to DCJ care.

Chapter Summary

Health and social care workers were dedicated and experienced professionals who wanted to make a difference in the women's lives that they provided care to. Many had worked in addiction for many years, which demonstrated their passion for the sector. These workers described stories of women caught up in a system that fails to meet the needs of women with SUDs, such as poor access to treatment, disenfranchised care and systemic stigma. Workers also described barriers to care that could make a difference, such as women accessing IPV support when it is offered and being more pro-active to address this problem.

CHAPTER NINE: PHASE THREE QUALITATIVE FINDINGS OF DEPARTMENT OF JUSTICE AND COMMUNITY WORKERS

Six perinatal DCJ workers donated their time to share their experiences working with pregnant women and new mothers with a history of IDU. All the DCJ staff interviewed were incredibly passionate about their work and wanted to make a difference. The interviews occurred in their workplace offices in four geographical areas in Sydney. Four women and two men were interviewed. All were qualified social workers and had been qualified from two years to over ten years. To maintain anonymity, gender-neutral pro-nouns are used through these findings. They were allocated a number instead of a pseudonym, as the pool of social workers employed directly to work in this space is small.

Theme 1: Contradictions in care

The DCJ workers, whose core business is child protection, acknowledged the challenges providing care to children without the consideration of the needs of the mother. Some workers spoke about having to choose and they reasoned that the child is the client, therefore they need to focus their attention on the child. For example, one worker said *'My role is not designed to be working with the parent and my role is child focused'* DCJ 5.

The different roles and responsibilities of professionals who worked with women across the health and community services sectors were acknowledged. This was not always conducive to working holistically. In the case of pregnancy family conferences (PFC), for example groups of health care and social welfare professionals are required to work together but were focused on different clients and perspectives.

> *'I suppose one of the other challenges is* [because]
> *we come from a child lens and lots of other services come from an adult lens. It's kind of that's also really challenging and obviously we need to work holistically. Like obviously child can't be safe, baby can't be safe without mum'.* DCJ 3

The child-focused lens of DCJ workers meant that the mothers' needs were not primary despite the interconnected nature of the health and welfare of the mother and child. One worker described a situation where they were at a PFC. All the workers knew about a mother's risk of escalating substance use, but she was not told. The worker felt that no one had thought to tell her as her client was not technically the mother, even though the mother's substance use affected the foetus.

This focus on the child meant that mothers did not receive the support from DCJ that they required. DCJ workers acknowledged that a child removal can be very traumatic for women. One of the issues as mentioned by DCJ workers was that counselling at this point was not routinely offered. Several DCJ workers noted that DCJ should have prepared mothers for all potential outcomes, including child removal, if this was a possible outcome.

The hope would be if that was going to happen, that we would have been having conversations that that's not the first time that they've heard that [child removal], *and especially this is the great thing about the pregnancy conferences, like those kinds of things get talk talked about throughout that.* DCJ 3

A different worker was asked if counselling was offered to mothers at the point of child removal. While the answer was no, they said that we should consider restoration as a matter of course.

'No, but do you know what it is? we should be thinking restoration as soon as you remove the child'. DCJ 1

There was an acknowledgment from this worker that, once the child is in care, the intensive support systems that were there during the pregnancy, 'will drop off' leaving the mother with much less support. This reduction in service provision was noted to be problematic by a DCJ worker who stated that women might be severely affected by this service gap:

'And they have another crisis point when babies are removed, that grief and loss goes through the roof. All those coping mechanisms that they were maybe working towards changing, but just couldn't quite get there, will end up in that exact same situation'. DCJ 4

The impact of the mother's situation on the child was acknowledged by DCJ workers and the impact on attachment.

'like if that's our bottom line, what does that mean for the attachment for the baby, and they're going to have to be separated [from] *them'.* DCJ 3

Theme 2: Treatment access

Arranging SUD treatment and housing for women in a timely manner, or at all, was frustrating for DCJ workers. DCJ workers described situations when services were full, long waiting lists for treatment centres, or no appropriate service was available. This was compounded if the mother was homeless, and one DCJ worker said that certain rehabilitation centres will not take a woman if she is homeless. In addition, a homeless woman did not have an address. Therefore, the rehabilitation centre could not determine what local government area they were from to ensure that they did not accept out of area requests.

DCJ workers described the challenges mothers faced accessing SUD treatment when children were removed into OOHC. Women wanted to be able to access treatment, but it was not always available. If there was a court order in place and a woman was required to access treatment services this could be extended if necessary and if treatment places were full. During this waiting period, other issues could arise. This is described in the following scenario:

> *This was not an ideal situation in many ways and also for the baby who whilst in care was developing attachments with other caregivers. The mother, who could not access rehab went to live with her aunt and unfortunately this was not a good scenario either as there was substance use within that family unit.* DCJ 4

Two other DCJ workers noted a similar scenario – that the mother could not access timely care, so the temporary care arrangement needed to be extended. One DCJ worker describes this situation as far from ideal.

> *'You know, a lot of our mums, things just don't align and so we also need to be mindful of not to set them up to fail'.* DCJ 3

Similarly, this DCJ worker acknowledged the challenges of mothers waiting for care, and the impact on attachment.

> *'Like if that's our bottom line, what does that mean for the attachment for the baby, and they're going to have to be separated* [from] *them'* DCJ 3

In addition to difficulties in accessing SUD treatment, one worker noted gaps in services that provide care to families. For example, some services that DCJ refer to, will only provide care when the mother still has custody of the child. One DCJ worker identified a time when a mother wanted to do a particular parenting course (as her child had autism), but this could not be funded as the child was in care.

'I guess because the services can't spend money on parents who may or may not have their children, even though they are still there parents and they still visit the children'. DCJ 6

Theme 3: Running into brick walls

DCJ workers described housing instability as a big issue for pregnant women and new mothers with SUDs. This created challenges for DCJ workers. For example, a pregnant woman may be placed in temporary housing within one local government area and be connected to a DCJ worker there. If she is then placed into more permanent accommodation or moves to temporary housing in a different area, the follow up could cease, as they are in another jurisdiction. Even more difficulties arise if the woman is from Interstate.

> *One problem with case managing someone in housing is the instability is of that difficulty to do with connection because they've been people moving around a lot. They can't access services and it services and services have boundaries as well. So then won't work with a client outside that locality.* DCJ 02

This DCJ worker was asked to elaborate on the complexities of people who move jurisdictions. For example, it was noted that sometimes a women will be followed up if they move from their jurisdiction to another, and they have their baby, but prenatally, many offices did not take transient people.

> *'A lot of our offices* [DCJ offices] *often don't take people moving around...we are the exception, we tend to, if they come into the area and they move out, we tend to still keep them. Just depends how far they move. Yeah. But the prenatally, um, you won't, a lot of offices won't'* DCJ 02

A different worker described how stressful it was for mothers who need housing. Sometimes, a woman can be in her last weeks of pregnancy and unable to secure housing.

> *'Well I had a mum like she, the week before* [she gave birth] *she was going from refuge to refuge. It was so stressful for her'* DCJ 4

According to DCJ workers, women were required to meet many expectations, which were difficult to adhere to at times. For example, one worker described a situation where a mother was asked to do drug urine screens by the court. To find a centre that would do this type of testing, she would have to travel up to an hour on a bus, pregnant.

> *'But if you live like in Coogee maybe it could take you an hour on the bus, or Eastern suburbs probably the hardest because you have to get to Kings Cross medical centre'.* DCJ 6

Other challenging situations for women include being directed to undertake parenting courses to prove to the authorities that they can parent. But if a woman does not have her child in her care, it isn't easy to put the learned skills into practice.

> *Like the court says you've got to do X, Y, and Zed or do these parenting courses or whatever, but they want you to have the child with you. So, you know, I've heard the frustration as well, fuck, you want me to do all this shit? But the um, "I need my child with me while I'm doing it and I need to be able to practice that".* DCJ 4

Theme 4: Changing child protection policy

DCJ workers stated that the goal is for the mother to parent and that this goal has shifted over time from removing children into care, to one of family preservation. Even if the baby was removed, one of the first conversations with a mother should be about restoration. DCJ workers want mothers to know that their goal was for women to parent their child. And that even if the baby was removed, many processes and supports can be provided to facilitate restoration, where possible. The following comment demonstrates this model of care.

> *'When I first meet, mum, [we say] our goal is for you to parent babies, even our language has changed...like our goals and is the same as yours, like how we get there, you know, that's what we need to work out, there are different ways, and our goal is for you to be able to parent bub'* DCJ 3

Another worker discussed that even when a baby is removed, it is now made clear to the mother that the goal is still for the child to be with their mother.

> *'So yeah, and at the hard thing is, especially if we go down the road of the parenting conference that babies do need to be placed outside the home...But we want to work on, like as I said, the goal is always for bub to go home.* DCJ 2

DCJ recognised that women often describe wanting their partners to be in their lives. This desire could be difficult to meet, especially if the partner needs support regarding substance use, or if they have mental health issues. It was mentioned that the care that DCJ provides mainly focuses on the baby, and the mother, but there is less support for the fathers. One worker felt that there needed to be more options focusing on family preservation to enable the father to be included. A case was discussed where one father had tried to get help for his SUD and found it difficult to access care, and so he threatened to commit suicide, all so he could access the care that he needed.

'Her partner was still using, but he was trying to sort himself out... and one of the things he did, which is so sad that's so intuitive, he threatened to commit suicide. So they scheduled him and he begged for them to keep him in until a bed became available at Rehab. DCJ 3

Theme 5: Trauma and Aboriginality, and service interactions

Nearly all of the DCJ workers had worked with Aboriginal mothers who, as they pointed out, had experienced significant levels of trauma at different points in their lives. In addition, the trauma and child protection issues and SUDs made for a more complex situation. While one worker commented that there were some extra options for Aboriginal people regarding support, they noted that this did not help too much when there was historical trauma.

'I think there are a few more options for Aboriginal people. Um, but that doesn't negate that trauma intergenerational trauma' DCJ 1

It was noted that child removal in Aboriginal families brings about a new level of trauma that is rooted in past governments policies on assimilation and the 'Stolen Generation'. One DCJ worker described a situation when they had been involved in a child removal that occurred straight from the hospital that included the police, and child protection workers. The DCJ worker mentioned that it was hard to bear witness to the grief experienced by this Aboriginal family.

'Well, look, the, the one that really sticks in my mind is with an Aboriginal mum at [one hospital], *and there were three generations of Aboriginal Women wailing, and police...*
So if you wanted to remake Rabbit Proof Fence in the Royal, it would have been good for it''
DCJ 03

Again, this trauma was described by a different worker who acknowledged the history of trauma in Aboriginal families and how this can impact experiences. This woman was a young first-time mother who went to gaol when she was pregnant and then had her child removed into care for several months while she went back into the prison system. The DCJ worker spoke about the difficulties that women in prison face when they have their babies removed, sometimes within 24-48 hours after giving birth.

In the prison system, literally within 24, 48 hours, they birth and they're out. So they're back there. They're handcuffed to beds. It's a really horrible experience for mums and then, you know, they go back to prison, they're lactating and their bodies are going through the changes but they don't have their little one. DCJ 4

This DCJ worker discussed the lack of culturally appropriate care when it comes to working with

Aboriginal families. For example, in one part of Sydney, she found an abundance of Aboriginal workers and Aboriginal services for Aboriginal people but not so much in other areas of Sydney. When she had encountered culturally appropriate services for Aboriginal people she felt that the outcomes were improved.

> *But I suppose the only, the one thing that really is lacking is in this area is working with Aboriginal families and Aboriginal mums. So you go out to Blacktown and it's amazing the services, the, you know, for Aboriginal mums…it just felt really right and then you come here in this particular pocket, it's really tricky to get that. DCJ 4*

And on top of this, it was noted that some Aboriginal services did not have Aboriginal staff.

> *Like even if you've got, um, an Aboriginal service, sometimes there's not…Aboriginal workers'* DCJ 04

Theme 6: Care delivery in the face of intimate partner violence

All the DCJ workers spoke about the difficulties of delivering services to women experiencing IPV. One worker stated that they found better outcomes for women when there was no man involved, as there was less IPV and, therefore, fewer complications. In addition, a male partner could pose a problem if he was still in active addiction. One worker commented:

> *'I also find…there is a really high success rate when there isn't a partner, and a really low success rate when there is a partner involved'* DCJ 05

When asked if domestic violence or substance use underpinned the outcome for these women, the DCJ worker replied that it was both. This DCJ worker was very experienced and having worked in the organisation for over ten years, however, they still find domestic violence very challenging to manage and difficult to mitigate risk. The presence of IPV also meant that it could be difficult to provide care. The needs of the women need to be balanced against the risk of IPV. When asked how they feel it is managed best, they sounded despondent.

> *It's really difficult…I've got to be really, really careful in protecting a woman, and being careful about the information provided. So, oh, generally I will interview a woman first, being very careful about the man…. um, we haven't solved that issue solved…I think we've got to come to grips and figure out community services fits with this. I know I keep on it the radar whole time…Um, to be able to get a man on board* [to make changes], *it's extremely difficult…it doesn't actually work to be honest.* DCJ 05

A different worker discussed the challenges they face when working with women encountering violence. They mentioned that there is a change in the underlying philosophy by DCJ on how IPV is managed. The responsibility to change the situation does not now rely solely on the mother, as she is the victim. It was mentioned that the men are the ones that need to make the change to improve the situation.

> *I suppose it's a little bit of a shift from how previously the work was, the onus, unfortunately was about the woman, you know, changing her behaviours and... But, there's still 'what can we do to make sure you and your unborn baby are safe and working more around that... I think in years gone by it's like, okay, she's not doing enough.* DCJ 03

This DCJ worker said that we need to harness the strengths that women display and focus on what is being done to keep their unborn child, or child safe, and then move forward from there. While at the same time acknowledging their roles as a worker in child protection and that they ultimately need to keep children safe.

> *'It's like, what, what is it that mum is doing, you know?... The child's in the room, they've got headphones on, the doors closed, or they're under the bed. I mean, not that that's going to keep a child safe, but we can work around, okay, mum is actually doing something'* DCJ 3.

Power and control were also mentioned as issues, not only in the context of men having power or control over women, but that this use of power is extended to DCJ workers who 'force' them to make changes in their lives or they will lose their child. One DCJ worker spoke of being upset at the injustices present in these women's lives.

> *'It's the feminist in me that tears at that one. This mum's being held accountable for something that's not her. Yeah* [fault]. *And they lose. They're the one that loses. A power and control continues because I'm controlling them'.* DCJ 2

Theme 7: Changing face of DCJ
Experiences that women have had with DCJ may be because of the historical reputation with DCJ and their own past experiences with DCJ. DCJ wants to change that reputation to make sure that women know that they are not there to remove their baby into care, but the goal is to work closely with the women, to build trust and support them wherever they are in their journey. Several of the workers spoke about a shift in how they work and how this can positively impact outcomes.

> *Just seeing,* [women] *being scared of engaging with services. Um, especially for families that have had previous involvement* [with DCJ] *and it hasn't been positive. Like, I think there has been a shift in the last couple of years. If you've had involvement, think they'll think it's DOCS.... and you know, I think even our persona in the public is, if even if you haven't had any contact with us, is that we remove children.* DCJ 3

This worker described that they feel that the reputation is slowly shifting, but not for everyone.

> *'I think we have a great relationship with* [the local hospital]...*and I think we've becoming a lot better at communicating and I think they're seeing that shift.. but still there is concern for some places that if they us information, it's going to be a knee jerk reaction of removal'* DCJ 3

Another worker described a similar experience, where they felt that some services were reluctant to report to DCJ as there was fear of what may happen if they did. The following comment demonstrates this:

> *I think there are still some services that are a bit resistant to telling family and community services information. We went out last week with a mum that had just given birth and she, um, she had been homeless, and she had admissions to mental health...we didn't get any information until she presented in hospital to have the baby* DCJ 4

This concern about the organisations reputation was echoed by another DCJ worker who voiced the following:

> *'Um, I guess the big things is the stigma that's attached to DCJ and the perception of that we're just going to steal children'* DCJ 6

One worker, who had been working in child protection for over five years, and who had worked under different sets of policies, felt that developing trust in clients who have had negative experiences with DCJ was important. One way to do this was to talk about these past experiences with their clients. This way they can talk about what can be done, and how they can achieve the client's goals.

> *'A lot of the families that I work with have had DCJ involvement previously and a lot of them had really bad experiences. And so I I talk with them about those experiences'* DCJ 1

In addition to developing trust, it was acknowledged that staff are now provided with higher levels of training, and there are better tools to aid decision making. It was identified that there was still some way to develop better pathways and collaborations with some smaller organisations.

> *'We now receive a lot of training, I think that's how I've been able to see a shift as well... like when I started three years ago to now, we are going through a lot of change at the moment and we've got a lot of training and our reforms policy and a law is changing'.* DCJ 1

Theme 8: So much work, so little time

DCJ workers discussed the difficulties of restoration and that at times it felt like they were facing an uphill battle. The time frames for restoration, or permanency have been shortened, providing less time for a woman to address issues. This is particularly challenging where grief due to the loss of a child is involved.

> *The court wants quick results. Now when I first came here, the court could take two years, now it could be over, five, six months. Um, so the court is asking for us to do... as soon as we remove a child, a plan for what's going to happen within two weeks... it's the beginning of the grief process, it's still, it's still that denial.* DCJ 1

It was suggested that when a child is removed and placed into OOHC, that support should be there to help the mother achieve restoration, which means providing lots of intensive support. However, the worker felt that the opposite occurred and that restoration was an uphill battle.

> *So, restoration is an uphill battle. It should be, and if you lose your job, for example, you should be getting support straight away to get a job back right? If you lose your child or for safety reasons your child is taken away, they deserve support both in terms of trauma and grief but also to get their child back.* DCJ 1

Restoration was not straightforward. The requirements that were in place for the women were difficult to meet. These were even more difficult to meet given the short amount of time that the courts stipulate. The repercussions of the grief associated with child removal as well as the complexities in these women's lives post child removal, are demonstrated in the following comment:

> 'It's too soon. But the court want it straight away, so we're dealing with the grief and they are probably going to use a crutch like um, a violent partner drugs or drugs or whatever else. Yeah. So it's a system that's set up to fail in terms of restoration'. DCJ 06

Theme 9: Building positive relationships

DCJ were really motivated to work closely with this group of families as the DCJ workers wanted to make a difference. They felt proud of their achievements and the relationships that they built with women. These relationships were built on developing trust and working tirelessly with mothers and their children to work towards providing positive outcomes. For example, one worker described a time when a young Aboriginal first-time mother using heroin was incarcerated. She gave birth in prison and her baby was removed into OOHC. The DCJ worker pushed and pushed and explored every avenue to seek restoration for this mother and her baby. She harnessed support of a team of

13 to be involved in her care. One worker even snuck baby clothes into the prison setting so the mother had the smell of her baby with her.

> *So I fought really hard...we went to the Supreme Court and we got a team around her and she's got another worker from the community restorative centre...just pushing because she was young and Aboriginal...she had a history of trauma and to separate from her child, her child from her, was just going to start off a whole...new level of trauma.* DCJ 4

This same worker discussed an issue where the trust levels broke down between her and the client mentioned in the scenario above. The DCJ worker felt disappointed in herself for not believing the mother, when she had been accused of using drugs out in the community.

> *'And I can still hear her voice because she, she could hear that, I took what they said for fact* [that she used drugs], *and she was upset and she's like, 'you didn't believe me'.* DCJ 4

Equally, when the time was not right for a woman to mother, this was respected, and mothers were informed that it was okay, if that was the case, but that did not mean that it could not happen later, if the situation changed. Importantly, the acknowledgement was made that it was more difficult as the baby was attached to another carer over time.

> *'Um, I think she just knew within herself that she didn't have the capacity at that point. Yeah. And you know, I always say to mums, you can always come back, you know, it may not be the right time right now and that's okay'.* DCJ 4

DCJ workers spoke about some recent success in re-uniting or keeping mothers and children together. Relationships between the DCJ workers and the mothers, were an important ingredient, and there was a positive reception to this new way of working. It was noted that when there is good communication, the fear of automatic child removal is allayed.

> *'To be able to work with someone and the fear kind of goes because there's this perception of DCJ and changing that we're working with them differently'* DCJ 5

The new way of working, according to DCJ, is a more transparent process, and promotes more positive relationships, according to one DCJ worker. They felt that being transparent with women made their job easier.

> *There's lots of positive outcomes. I think, um, if they have this level of trust, which I like to try and establish early, um, it's much easier to work together... I think because we like to be a bit more transparent than we used to be, I can very, very honest pretty quickly sort of gain a rapport.* DCJ 1

Being transparent overall, made it easier for DCJ workers to have discussions with women who were going to have infants or children removed into care. Additionally, they did not have to tell the mother what they wanted to hear, but instead, clear and honest discussions could be had.

> *I suppose a lot of times they will them what they want to hear and enable that* [previously]. *But when we can all be honest, you can plan and we can tell clients that if things go wrong we can still plan. Doesn't mean your baby's going to be coming into care. So I'm pretty quick on talking about babies coming into care, or not.* DCJ 1

Mothers informed of their baby's removal before birth were less likely to wonder why DCJ were there. While DJ workers recognised this as a problematic situation, it was regarded as less traumatic.

> *'They knew exactly what was happening. So although like it wasn't an outcome that they wanted, it made that process a lot, so much smoother. There was no crisis of DCJ running to the hospital'.* DCJ 2

Chapter Summary

The DCJ workers were highly passionate and dedicated professionals who wanted to make a difference in the lives of the women they worked with. At times they were constrained with what they could do due to high workloads and limited resources. They also recognised the limitations of what they could provide for women, as ultimately, they worked in child protection, and the child was their client. Barriers to the provision of good care for women, as described by the DCJ workers, were IPV. Other barriers were lack of support for women after child removal and the lack of focus on assisting the father

CHAPTER TEN: PHASE FOUR DISCUSSION

This is the first known Australian study that identifies health care experiences and needs of pregnant women and new mothers who are current injecting drug users. Thirteen women who are typically hard to reach and under-represented in research, policy and planning (Biondi et al., 2020, Topp et al., 2013) were allowed to voice their needs and experiences and insights into how they perceived care. The women's voices are central to this research, and highlight needs from their perspective so that health and social systems can respond in ways that are acceptable to these populations of women (Islam et al., 2012). This study is strengthened through a mixed methodology design where perspectives from care providers are included as well as standardised quantitative measures of women, thus providing a more comprehensive overview of the situation to seek the 'truth'.

Multiple and complex issues that exacerbated the already challenging lives faced by women with SUDs were highlighted in this study. Transience, homelessness, high rates of mental health disorders, violence, and trauma were common for interviewed women. Additionally, power imbalances left women frustrated, and women described living in a world that was setting them and their children up to fail. Yet, within all this, women explored ideas of hope and determination. This section sought to provide insights and explanations for the situations faced by women through the integration of data from Phase 1 to Phase 3.

This study had three aims. The first was to determine the health and psychosocial needs and experiences of pregnant women and women who have recently given birth and are current injecting drug users in NSW, Australia. The second aim was to provide important insights into how these women perceive health and social support, their experiences of accessing it and how it may or may not address their health and social needs. The third aim was to examine how service providers can best support, plan and deliver appropriate evidence-based care to meet the needs of these women.

This study captured how these women navigate pregnancy, hospitals, primary health care services, SUD treatment and rehabilitation services. It also documented their interactions with staff, including doctors, midwives, nurses and DCJ workers. In addition, this study detailed women's health and social care needs and answered the following research questions:

For pregnant women and new mothers who inject drugs:

1. What services, including both pregnancy and non-pregnancy services, are available?
2. What guidelines are available to support this group of women?

3. What are the current health and psychosocial status of these women?

4. What are the health and psychosocial needs of these women?

5. What are the health service experiences and interactions of these women?

This chapter presents a brief overview of the research findings. These are then discussed in relation to the current literature, gaps in knowledge and implications for policy and practice.

The context of pregnant and parenting women with SUD

The systematic review undertaken as part of the background for this study (chapter 2) identified that many women did not fully engage in health care for fear of being found out that they were 'drug users'; and that their children would be removed into care. Women wanted more autonomy and choice in treatment options and felt stigmatised within health systems. In addition, there was a lack of suitably available treatment for women and their children, resulting in a lack of access and uptake of care. Furthermore, some women lacked the personal funds and financial aid to access treatment. This was mainly found in the USA, where most studies were conducted, and universal health care is unavailable, and health care access is limited

According to women, the benefits of SUD treatment included learning parenting skills and enjoying the day-to-day routine that treatment afforded (Eindbinder, 2009). However, some women found they were powerless to make decisions about their own health needs and their children's needs (Demirci et al., 2015, Gueta, 2017). This sense of powerlessness resulted in the perception that their parenting abilities were undermined.

A review of services for pregnant women and new mothers with SUDs within NSW identified nine specialist residential rehabilitation services, with six of these in Sydney and three in regional areas. These programs varied in length of time, whether they take women on OAT and the maximum age of children allowed in services. All appear to be affordable and low cost. However, long waiting lists to access these residential services are common, and there is no one-size-fits-all model. A range of interventions are offered, including counselling, cognitive behavioural therapy, parenting courses underpinned by attachment theory, and domestic violence counselling.

Of the 15 local health districts in NSW, 12 have specialist pregnancy services, and eight of these are in Sydney or Greater Sydney, which includes the Illawarra, the Blue Mountains and the Central Coast. However, there are no specialist services for pregnant women with SUDs for those living in Far Western NSW, Western NSW and Southern NSW, indicating a gap in care for women in these regions. In addition, two centres were identified that provide day only services for women, including care for pregnant women and new mothers with SUD. One service is located in the Blue Mountains, and another is in inner-city Sydney.

Australian clinical guidelines for the care of pregnant women with a history of IDU meet the WHO recommendations. Only two Australian guidelines, the national and the NSW Health guidelines as well as the WHO guidelines highlight the importance of culturally appropriate care for Aboriginal women. This approach should be central to all Australian guidelines. Culturally appropriate care is a key health strategy for closing the health gap between Aboriginal and non-Aboriginal Australians and has the potential to reduce inequalities in health care access and improve the quality and effectiveness of care for Aboriginal people (Laverty et al., 2017).

The guideline review identified the need for all women to be screened for substance use as early as possible during the antenatal period. Tailored psychosocial interventions and referral to an appropriate multidisciplinary drug and alcohol management program should be undertaken. In addition, further education of staff is recommended regarding the provision of specialised care. Women should be encouraged to breastfeed, including women on OAT, unless the risks outweigh the benefits. Babies with NAS should be cared for using guidelines such as Neonatal Abstinence Syndrome Guidelines (NSW Health, 2013, QLD Health, 2021). Additional recommendations include the need for continuity of care and discussing sudden infant death syndrome, tobacco use and contraception. Screening should occur for mental health issues and IPV, care should be delivered with a trauma-informed care focus, and stigma should be addressed through awareness training.

The needs and experiences of women in NSW

Thirteen women with a recent history of injecting drug use were interviewed during pregnancy and up to a year after giving birth. Findings indicated that the women interviewed in this current study were highly marginalised with multiple unmet health and psychosocial needs. Many were engaged in heavy substance use, with six women injecting at least daily up to three months preceding the primary interview. Almost all were dependent on opiates, with 11 women on OAT. Women had high levels of self-reported mental health diagnosis and over half (7/13) exhibited some distress on the EDPS. None of the eligible women were on contraception, six were overdue for a cervical screen, and five reported having untreated hepatitis C.

All women relied on government income, had limited social support, and most (11/13) had other children living in out of home care. Nearly all women (12/13) had experienced recent IPV. The trauma of having children placed in OOHC and IPV left the women traumatised. Five women identified as Aboriginal.

Women reported feeling abandoned and let down by the systems designed to assist them. They described feeling powerless, continuously surveyed, and service providers questioned their ability to mother, despite the fact that the mothers felt generally confident in their own parenting abilities. Women felt that they were constantly being set up to fail, and no matter what they did, it was just not good enough. Women also spoke about the sadness and guilt resulting from their substance use and its impact on their children. Yet, despite the challenges, women desired to parent their children, had hope for the future, and valued positive relationships and experiences with care providers.

The experiences of health, social care and DCJ providers caring for women with a history of injecting drug use

Thirteen health and social care workers were interviewed. These participants were: four nurses, three midwives, two doctors, two social workers, a social work student and a rehabilitation manager. All appeared to be passionate and dedicated professionals who advocated for positive outcomes for their clients. However, workers described many difficulties working in this space. They described the sector as stigmatised and underfunded, and care that was fragmented. In addition, there were challenges to managing the complex needs of women with many competing priorities, including SUD, IPV, mental health disorders and underlying trauma.

Six perinatal DCJ workers who work specifically with pregnant women and new mothers with SUDs were qualified social workers who described being passionate and motivated to make a difference. They reported challenges such as care priorities, difficulties getting women into timely treatment, and barriers to providing suitable housing for women. The DCJ workers frequently spoke about the new policies that focused on restoration where possible, as opposed to historical policies that aligned with the removal of children (DCJ, 2021a). They hoped that new policies would improve outcomes for women and their public reputation which they felt was tarnished.

Data analysis: Meta themes

This study's final data analysis stage involved integrating the separate phases of quantitative and qualitative results (inferences) into coherent and meaningful 'meta-inferences' or themes (Onwuegbuzie and Combs, 2010). The data were integrated using a table, to identify key findings, themes, and areas requiring further exploration, using the 'following a thread' method (Moran-Ellis et al., 2006), as described in the methods chapter. Once the meta themes were identified they were reviewed alongside the socioecological model. Each meta theme was allocated a corresponding component of the socioecological model which provided a framework for the analysis. The meta themes were examined alongside key findings from the quantitative data, the situational analysis and the guideline review to generate a multi-faceted overview of the situation. Finally, these meta-themes were discussed in relation to recent literature in the field, and the implications of policy and practice and recommendations discussed.

Meta-theme and socioecological model relationship

Following the integration of the data, four meta-themes were identified. These themes were: self-determination, trauma- with the sub-themes of IPV and OOCH, power and stigma and finally, systemic challenges. Self-determination pairs with the 'individual' component of the socioecological model. This relates to women's internal drive to mother their children, be housed, have stability, and live a resemblance of a 'normal life'. This theme also includes sadness and guilt for their own mistakes and how this has influenced outcomes. Its paired 'individual' component relates to individual characteristics such as demographic and mental health influence outcomes and factors impeding their ability to parent.

A woman's trauma is paired with the 'interpersonal and relationship' component of the socioecological model. The trauma associated with IPV and OOHC meant that women presented with fear of past and current violence and unresolved grief. Women's relationships with health and social care providers are critical to quality care. Trauma is paired with the 'interpersonal and relationship' component as women's trauma is related to relationships and interactions with partners and care providers, such as DCJ.

Power and stigma are paired with the 'organisational and community' component of the socioecological model. Women described power imbalances and stigma within systems, which meant that women were sometimes afraid to come forward for care. The 'organisational and community' component explores settings, such as health care and social services, where power imbalances and stigma occur.

The final meta-theme was systemic challenges, paired with 'policy' on the socioecological model. This relates to women's barriers and challenges within medicalised health care and a stringent social welfare system. It is paired with 'policy' as this examines broad societal factors that create a climate that makes it difficult for women to access appropriate and timely care such as SUD treatment and appropriate housing.

I have chosen to represent these relationships as a Venn diagram (see Diagram 4), rather than the traditional socioecological model depicted in chapter three to illustrate how the layers of the socioecological model are interconnected and inextricably linked. Women's experiences occur within and across the layers of the four layers of the socioecological model. Moreover, they are dynamic, influenced, and influenced by each other. For example, stigma impacts service access, influencing DCJ decisions on whether a woman can keep her baby.

etween the meta-themes and the socioecological model

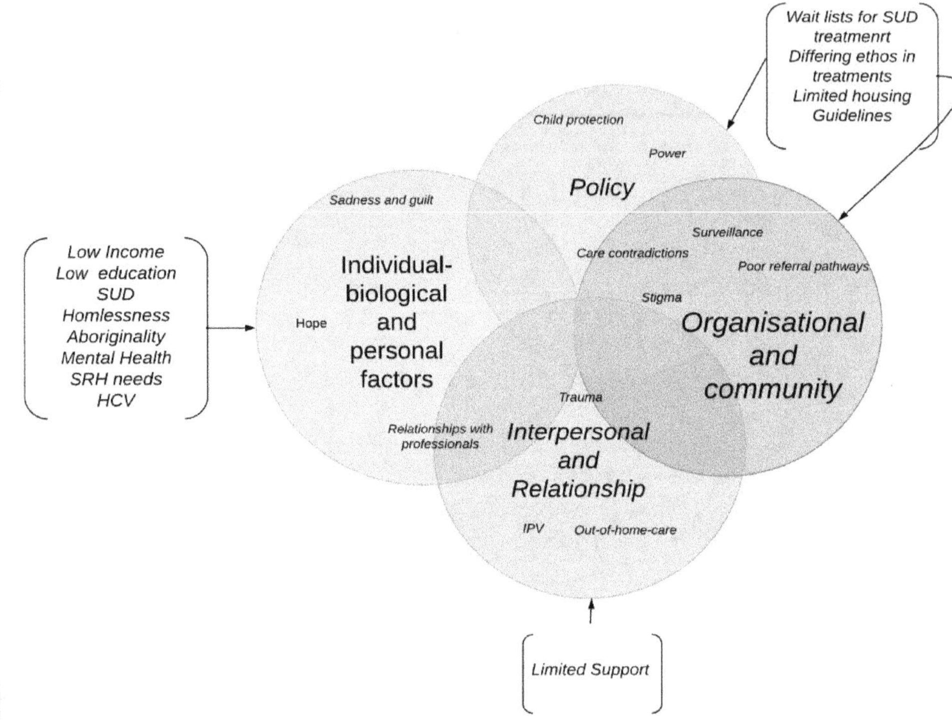

e

n n=13	Health and social care workers n=13	DCJ workers n=6	Service review	Guideline Summary	Meta inference
social efits as e 10 years	**1. Stigma** 1.1 Stigma working in the area of addiction 1.2 Affects funding burnout 1.3 Stigma on women by other staff	**1. Contradictions in care** 1.1 There for the child, not the mother 1.3 Recognition this can be an issue 1.4 mothers not offered counselling for OOHC	9 specialist residential rehabilitation services in NSW, 6 are in Sydney. 12 of 15 LHDs have specialist pregnancy services.	1. All women should be screened for substance use in antenatal care. Self-report of use of substances may be more valuable than UDS	Self determinat
ere in a ationship d using e- 6/13	**2. Competing priorities** 2.1 Women are burnout, have such high demands placed on them, (e.g. multiple appts, OAT)	**2. Treatment access** 2.1 Hard to access timely treatment 2.3 Led to extension temporary care arrangement 2.4 Baby in care longer – bonds with other carers	Two day only services exist Vary in the length of time. Not all take OAT women on OAT,	2. Psychosocial interventions with SUD and referral to a drug and alcohol management program should occur. Further training of staff is recommended 3. Pregnant women who use ATS and cocaine should be advised to cease. Those dependent on opioids	Trauma: Relationships OOHC IPV
t sed – 11 o women men en had d MH ing at distress	**3. Access to care** 3.1 Hard to get access to good MH care 3.2 Need trauma-informed care 3.3 Lack of recognition re: MH- the SUD is blame 3.1 No one size fits all	**3. Running into brick walls** 3.1 Housing instabilities 3.2 Moving jurisdictions and not being followed up 3.3 Unrealistic expectation	The ages of children allowed in services vary. All low cost. Waiting lists to access residential services can be long.	should commence on OAT. Pregnant women who use BZDs should be transferred to a long-acting BZD 4. No pharmacological treatment is available for ATS, cannabis, or cocaine 5. Women should be encouraged to breastfeed 6. Babies with NAS should be cared for using other	Power and stig

...men Quan n=13	Health and social care workers n=13	DCJ workers n=6	Service review	Guideline Summary	Meta int...
...men had self-...rted HCV ...women ...ded on-time ...f the eligible 10 ...en was on ...raception ...women ...due for CST	**4. Child removal and inconsistent care** 4.1 removals were inconsistent 4.2 Difficult to follow women up as they are disengaged, and not their job 4.3 Distressing for both women and staff 4.4 Causes more trauma	**4 Changing child protection policy** 4.1 Goal to mother 4.2 Negative public view 4.3 Potential to include fathers 4.4 Women are traumatised from past policies	There are a breadth of services are provided which include counselling, CBT, TC, IPV counselling, parenting courses and harm reduction in some	guidelines such as Neonatal Abstinence Syndrome Guidelines (NSW Health, 2013) 7. In addition: Competent care must be practiced for Aboriginal women. Continuity of care should be practiced. The following should be discussed: sleeping practices, sudden infant death syndrome (SIDS) and tobacco and contraception. In addition, screening should occur for mental health issues and IPV. Care should be delivered with a trauma-informed care focus, and stigma should be addressed through awareness training.	Systemi...
...of 47 children ...ether, 37 in ...C ...: 9/13 risk ...l isolation ...: 10/13 women ...ed high	**5. Falling through the cracks** 5.1 Missing care provision for children 2-5 years 5.2 Limited appropriate care, e.g., playgroups 5.3 Lack of follow up care 5.4 Structural barriers	**5. Trauma and Aboriginality** 5.1 Systemic trauma 5.2 Historical trauma and OOHC 5.2 Need better culturally appropriate care			
...: 5/13 women ...ed high on the ...	**6. Power** 6.1 HCW over women 6.2 DCJ workers over women 6.3 Different opinions 6.4 Undermined by DCJ who have the power	**6. Care in the face of intimate violence** 6.1 Very difficult to address 6.2 A main reason for OOHC			
...DV screening: ...women were ...d of their ...ners	**7. Violence** 7.1 One of the biggest challenges 7.2 Women have lost faith 7.3 Some women lie about it 7.4 Reason why children in OOHC 7.5 Mothers do better with no man	**7. Changing face of FACS** 7.1 Old reputation influences outcomes			
	8. Mothers determination 8.1 Women have enormous strength 8.2 Women have hope	**8. So much work, so little time** 8.1 Little time to change situations			

uan n=13	Health and social care workers n=13	DCJ workers n=6	Service review	Guideline Summary	Meta inferenc
	8.2 Empowerment works	8.2 New timeframes =more pressures			
		9. Building positive relationships 9.1 Passionate 9.2 Motivated to make change 9.3 Transparency 9.4 new ways of working			

The following section describes the findings of each meta-theme and their alignment to the socioecological model. This section is divided into four sections, each comprising one meta-theme. Finally, the implications for policy and practice will be discussed, and a model of practice that is acceptable to the client population will be recommended.

Meta-theme 1: Individual- self-determination

> 'Yeah, and I was able to just have my little bonding time with him. We build a nice strong bond'

This discussion places the needs of the woman at the centre. Most discourse that surrounds women who are pregnant or mothers with SUDs, revolves around the protection of the child, and often this is at the expense of the woman's needs. Furthermore, this discourse perpetuates the good mother-bad mother dichotomy of mothers that cannot care for their children (Meyers et al., 2021). Therefore, we must explore the possibility of a differing world view that considers the opinions and needs of pregnant or parenting women living in highly challenging contexts (Dunkerley, 2017). This meta-theme will discuss women's desire and determination to mother and the individual characteristics that impede a woman's ability to self-determination.

Determination to mother

Women in this study faced significant challenges to be a 'good mother' such as addiction, mental health issues, poverty and limited social support. Marginalisation, chronicity of SUDs, and long histories of mental health combined with underlying trauma and IPV exacerbated these issues. Despite the challenges, women displayed strength, resilience, hope, and determination to parent their children, even when not in their care. Women overall were optimistic about their future. They wanted a 'normal life' and, for some, a nuclear family, even when violence was present.

Alongside women's feeling of hope were high levels of parenting confidence with ten out of 13 women scoring high on the KPCS. These findings suggest that their belief in their ability to parent successfully was high (Bandura et al., 1999). This offers a different narrative to the bad-mother identity perpetuated by the broader society (Harvey et al., 2015). Parental self-efficacy (PSE), as is measured in the KPCS, is a key factor that relates to maternal depression, stress and child development (Jones and Prinz, 2005). Mothers with high PSE generally have lower rates of depression, and conversely, the opposite is true (Pontoppidan et al., 2019). However, in this PhD results were mixed and three women with low KPCS scores, had high distress and depression scores on the EPDS and four women with high KPCS scores, also had high distress and depression scores on the EPDS. This may be due to high background levels of mental health disorders which may have confounded the overall KPCS results.

Research on PSE and women with SUDs is scant (Zand et al., 2017, Chou et al., 2018). There is a gap in the literature regarding PSE among mothers receiving SUD treatment and who have mental health disorders (Matsuda et al., 2019). High KPCS scores in this study may be because many women already had children and possess experiential knowledge vital for PSE (Pontoppidan et al., 2019). Additionally, many women undertook attachment-based parenting courses within residential rehabilitation settings. These courses can empower women by enhancing mental health; self-esteem; parenting confidence and competence (Zhang and Bennett, 2003).

Parenting programs should include motivational interviewing that harness the internal drive of women (Ingersoll et al., 2013, Karatay et al., 2010). Programs that are underpinned by attachment theory that address a mother's emotional dysregulation to increase maternal sensitivity (Dakof et al., 2010, Suchman et al., 2010) should be initiated as early as possible, preferably in the first semester of pregnancy as this timepoint presents a unique opportunity for change (Chou et al., 2018). These programs can positively affect substance use, mental health, parenting practices, and family functioning (Dakof et al., 2010, Suchman et al., 2010).

One program offered at the nine residential rehabilitation centres that holds promise for mothers with SUDs is the Parenting Under Pressure (PUP) program. This attachment-based program includes a component on emotional regulation by using mindfulness. A recent randomised controlled trial of the PUP program versus treatment as usual from the UK, found that the PUP program significantly reduced child abuse potential and improved parental emotional regulation (Barlow et al., 2019). This program has demonstrated positive effects on mothers using methadone (Dawe et al., 2003), and those involved in the child protection system (Dawe, 2008). Mindfulness in mothers with SUDs is an emerging area. More research is needed, with larger samples to allow for further refinement of programs and approaches to support families with complex issues (Dawe et al., 2021).

Positively, seven of the nine reviewed residential rehabilitation programs offer parenting programs underpinned by attachment theory (two were unknown). Most women in this current study (10/13) had undertaken parenting courses once their baby was born, indicating earlier support could prove more useful for these women. Although DCJ workers noted that for women without custody of their children, there was no opportunity to apply new skills.

The positivity and high levels of PSE among women were intersected by deficit models of child protection and medicalised health care systems that provide limited opportunities to address the multiple complexities women face (Russ et al., 2020). Despite these challenges, many women were able to 'hold it together' (Marcellus, 2017), while they often met multiple demands simultaneously. These demands include attending residential rehabilitation, DCJ meetings, parenting classes, counselling, medical appointments, and ceasing or reducing drug use. The recognition of these strengths is important and can lead to better relationships between women and caseworkers (Fusco, 2019). The implementation of strengths-based programs can reduce substance use and improve mental health, parenting practices, and family functioning (Dakof et al., 2010). Strength-based programs may also mitigate the guilt felt by mothers by acknowledging the impact of substance use (Smith, 2006). Recognition of guilt can increase maternal-infant bonding (Rockefeller et al., 2019).

Breastfeeding
Breastfeeding for women with SUDs, including mothers on OAT should be encouraged for at least six months (WHO and UNICEF, 2003). It was recommended in all reviewed guidelines, apart from the RANZCOG and NDARC guidelines, where it was omitted. Breastfeeding improves maternal-infant bonding, attachment and maternal sensitivity (Ainsworth, 1985), and can decrease symptoms in babies with NAS (Holmes et al., 2017, Wu and Carre, 2018).

Promisingly, six women in this study did breastfeed. Although it is not known how long they continued to breastfeed for, the women indicated that it was only for a short time, such as the baby's first week of life. For two women, this was interrupted due to child-removal within a week of birth. Low rates of breastfeeding in mothers with SUD have been found in Australian and overseas studies. In Australia, Abdel-Latif et al. (2013) conducted a retrospective audit of mothers with SUDs discharged from maternity units and found only 333 of 879 (32%) of mothers breastfed their infants at discharge. In comparison to 86% of other mothers, these rates are low. Breastfeeding rates in a study from the USA reported even lower rates (Yonke et al., 2018).

Interviewed health care and social care providers noted that early cessation of breastfeeding was an issue, especially if a baby was removed into OOHC. For women who wanted to breastfeed their babies in OOHC, some staff felt women did not deserve to do so. Positively, the newly updated Australian National Breastfeeding Strategy supports women with children in OOHC to breastfeed, with support through a lactation consultant and child protection workers (COAG, 2019). Despite these recommendations, midwives interviewed for this study said that in their experience, DCJ workers made it difficult for women to continue to breastfeed and did not facilitate care.

Given the low breastfeeding rates among women with SUDs, further research is warranted to understand the breastfeeding decisions of women with and without babies in their care and to clarify the context for professionals who support these women. For example, the literature review noted that women were concerned that they may pass methadone or HCV onto their baby (Demirci et al., 2015). There is a dearth of literature of breastfeeding for women with babies in OOHC (Blythe et al., 2021). One Swedish study found low rates of breastfeeding in foster children at four months of age compared to a control group (10% vs 31%). However, it is unclear if these lower rates were attributable to other factors such as low socioeconomic status. (Köhler et al., 2015). Another study from Australia interviewed 184 foster carers on their views of mothers breastfeeding their children in foster care (Blythe et al., 2021). Foster carers noted concerns about the safety of breastmilk from substance use and questioned the value of breastfeeding if reunification was not possible. Some carers even discarded expressed breastmilk and limited contact with mothers (Blythe et al., 2021). Conversely, breastfeeding was viewed positively if reunification was the goal, demonstrating that more education and support for foster mothers is required so that mothers can continue to breastfeed (Blythe et al., 2021).

Importantly and while research is limited, breastfeeding has been associated with lower rates of child abuse. A prospective Australian study of 6000 women and their children, examined substantiated child maltreatment cases over 15 years (Strathearn et al., 2009). This study found that even when they adjusted for confounding factors such as economic status, children who were not breastfed or were breastfed for less than four months were 2.6 times more likely to be neglected by their mothers than children breastfed for four months or more (Strathearn et al., 2009). A different study from the USA analysed outcomes of 4,159 adolescents from the National Longitudinal Study of Adolescent to Adult Health Study. This study found that for adolescents who were never breastfed, compared to adolescents breastfed for nine months, there were reduced odds of having experienced neglect (odds ratio=0.54) and sexual abuse (OR = 0.47) (Kremer and Kremer, 2018).

These findings indicate that breastfeeding may offer a protective role regarding child abuse and neglect, but this is an under-researched area. Further research is required to establish a causal link between breastfeeding and the reduction in abuse and neglect (Kremer and Kremer, 2018). In addition, promoting breastfeeding is relatively simple and inexpensive and can strengthen the relationship between a woman and her baby, and include benefits such as a contraceptive effect

(Kennedy and Visness, 1992). These studies do not mention mothers with illicit substance use, so the relationship between breastfeeding and child abuse and neglect in this cohort is unknown.

Child abuse potential

This current study found that six mothers had indicators for child abuse when they completed the BCAP, indicating their determination to mother is at risk. Four of these six women did not have children in their care, suggesting that the BCAP may be relevant for this population. In addition, there were correlations with other risk factors for child abuse, such as high rates of mental health issues, stress and limited support, which must be taken into account (Begle et al., 2010). While it is known that women with SUDs are at higher risk of child abuse (Walsh et al., 2003, Grella et al., 2006), the mechanism in which this occurs is less precise with studies reporting similar rates of abuse when compared to peers from similar social and demographic backgrounds (Hogan et al., 2006, Kepple, 2018). Four of the six women found to have indicators for child abuse did not have children in their care, indicating that the BCAP may be relevant for this population. In addition, there were correlates with other risk factors for child abuse, such as high rates of mental health issues and limited support, which must be taken into account.

Mitigating risks and decreasing child abuse and neglect underpin child protection policy worldwide (Dawe et al., 2017). One of the tools used in NSW when making decisions regarding the welfare of a child is called a Structured Decision Making (SDM) tool. This empirically-based actuarial risk assessment provides a score that indicates the probability of harm based on a list of predictors associated with child maltreatment (Barlow et al., 2012). The SDM can provide precise, probabilistic estimates of maltreatment however, like any risk assessment, it can produce false negative or false positive results (AIFS, 2022). One measure proposed by Dawe et al. (2017) is using the BCAP alongside the SDM, which may be useful for further assessing abuse potential in mothers with SUDs. The use of the BCAP can provide additional information on a women's capacity to parent, and a high score can signal that more support is required (Dawe et al., 2017). The addition of this instrument may be helpful for DCJ workers, as this thesis found that decision making, especially whether to remove a child or not, played heavily on their minds which was linked to burnout and stress. In addition, and with further training, the BCAP can be utilised by other staff supporting women including midwives, nurses and family and childhood nurses (Ellonen et al., 2019).

Challenges to self-determination: homelessness and mental health
Being able to 'hold it together' for women in this study depended on external factors such as their personal and professional support and if basic human rights such as safety, a home, and the ability to live free of violence were met. When access to these external factors was challenged, some women were close to or at breaking point. They became frustrated, angry, overwhelmed, and felt set up to fail. These perceptions were corroborated by both health and social care providers and DCJ workers, who highlighted failures in many aspects of care. This includes failures in relational care such as a breakdown in client-professional relationships, shifting notions of trust, and feeling undermined within health and child protection systems that are both inflexible and punitive (Russ et al., 2020, Bryant et al., 2022). When basic needs such as appropriate housing are not met, this can derail women further. Housing insecurity and homelessness in women in this study were common, demonstrating a significant gap in resource availability.

The link between homelessness, mental health, and substance use for women is well-known (Flatau, 2021). Compared to housed women, women experiencing homelessness are at risk of cardiovascular disease and respiratory diseases (Teruya et al., 2010), increased violence and STIs (Caton et al., 2013), and mortality rates up to ten times higher (Cheung and Hwang, 2004). Homelessness in pregnancy is linked to adverse perinatal outcomes, such as preterm birth, low birth weight neonates, neonatal intensive care admission, and delivery complications (DiTosto et al., 2021).

Four women in this study experienced homelessness which is appalling and signals the extreme marginalisation of these women. Very little data exists on pregnancy and homelessness both internationally, and in Australia (Murray et al., 2018, DiTosto et al., 2021), as a result the true extent of these issues are unknown (Murray et al., 2018). There is no comprehensive data collection. Data is only collected where pregnant homeless women may present, such as at domestic violence services, hospitals or antenatal care.

Residential treatment settings were identified as 'home' for many women in this study. While this respite for women it is temporary and retaining a place relies on engagement in programs and abide by the rules and codes of conduct. If these are compromised, women can be involuntarily discharged demonstrating that systems are not fully equipped to meet the needs of women with challenging requirements and that more support such as education and skills development using a trauma-focused framework are required (Marcellus, 2014).

Mental health was a huge issue and challenge for women interviewed for this study. Nearly all women stated they had a mental health disorder and over half of the women had a positive EDPS score of at least 10. While these findings must be viewed with caution, as four women were screened using the EDPS outside the recommended period of pregnancy to 12 weeks post-delivery, the rate of mental health disorders in this study appears higher than in other similar studies. One Australian study that retrospectively examined medical charts of 879 drug-dependent mother NSW and the ACT found that psychiatric comorbidity was identified in 45% of the women reviewed (Oei et al., 2009). Compared to other groups of Australian women without SUDs, rates of mental health disorders are much lower. One study found rates of distress in women experiencing IPV were 8.1%, and rates of distress in women with DCJ involvement were 8.1% (Khanlari et al., 2019).

Discrepancies were found in this study for self-reported mental health versus the EPDS for all five Aboriginal women. All Aboriginal women stated they had a mental health condition but did not score high on the EPDS. This is a typical result for Aboriginal women where the tool it is yet to be validated (Kotz et al., 2021). Cultural and literacy issues, mistrust of mainstream services or fear of consequences of identified depression may contribute to responder bias (Austin and Highet, 2017). Novel screening tools for Aboriginal women are required so we can better identify and respond to depressive symptoms in the perinatal period (Kotz et al., 2016). The Kimberly Mums Mood Scale (KMMS) has been found to be an effective tool for Aboriginal women at risk of anxiety and depressive disorders (Kotz et al., 2016). This tool was developed by and for women living in the remote Kimberly region of Western Australia, which is a version EPDS Similar tools need to be designed for Aboriginal women living in other settings so that interventions and support can occur in a timely manner.

Health, social care, and DCJ workers were challenged regarding working with women with mental health issues. Disentangling substance use from the mental health issues from the trauma proved difficult and providers were frustrated when women would not access referrals for care. The literature review suggested that having a peer with similar experiences can mitigate the effects of access barriers and limited supportive network (Kuo et al., 2013) and this model utilised SUD programs. Furthermore, there are no validated screening tools specifically for depression and anxiety women with SUDs and this is an area that requires urgent review (Arnaudo et al., 2017). Similarly, there is a need for improved evidence-based interventions for these women (Oei et al., 2009).

Challenges to self-determination: competing health priorities

Women had to prioritise care and meet multiple and competing demands and therefore, several health issues fell to the bottom of 'the list'. Women in this current study had low rates of CST screening and untreated HCV infection. Little is known about the rates of cervical cancers in women who use illicit drugs (Kricker et al., 2013). However, one Australian data linkage study found that illicit drug use was independently associated with a lower incidence of cervical screening and an increased risk of CIN 2/3, a risk factor for cancerous cells on the cervix (Kricker et al., 2013).

Low rates in interviewed women is interesting as cervical screening is safe in any stage of pregnancy and recommended for women who are overdue (Cancer Council, 2019). It is possible women were not screened as stated by women, or they were screened during routine antenatal care but were unaware this occurred. Both scenarios are problematic (Cancer Council, 2019). Promisingly, Australia will be one of the first countries to offer self-collection through GP settings to all women through the National Cervical Screening Program (DoH, 2019). This is an important initiative acceptable to vulnerable and under screened populations who may benefit through targeted health promotion and education (Saville et al., 2018). Cervical screening in GP settings can be provided by nurses as well as doctors and this has been demonstrated to improve rates of screening through a targeted follow up and recall approach (Rennie et al., 2015). Furthermore, screening rates have been down nationally due to Covid-19, so catch-up is still underway. Future impacts of lower screening rates due to Covid-19 are unknown (Bu and Morgan, 2021).

Treatment for HCV is not recommended in pregnancy or breastfeeding but is recommended at any other stage. Four out of five women in this PhD who had HCV, were eligible for treatment. They were in rehabilitation at the time, which is a perfect opportunity that was missed. Direct-acting antiviral therapies for HCV are highly effective and 95% of people can achieve viral clearance, having clear benefits from a public health perspective (Read et al., 2017, The Kirby Institute, 2019). The situational analysis only identified one rehabilitation setting that offered hepatitis C treatment. Barriers to treatment in these settings include access to a GP who can prescribe under the highly specialised (s100) program. One model to overcome this barrier to care is through the use of nurse practitioners. Nurse practitioners work at an advance level of practice and can diagnose and prescribe medications within their speciality field (Ling, 2009). From April 2021 nurse practitioners are eligible to prescribe hepatitis B and hepatitis C treatments under the s100 program. Another model, which is more feasible considering there are limited numbers of nurse practitioners in Australia (1556 in 2017) is a nurse-led outreach model supported by s100 prescribing medical practitioners. Nurse led models of care have found that HCV treatment can provided safely and efficiently (Overton et al., 2019). Expansion of care is an important component of the strategy to eliminate HCV infection as a public health concern by 2030 (Overton et al., 2019). Treatment in PHC facilities is also an acceptable model for treatment (Read et al., 2017).

Findings from this meta-theme demonstrated that women wanted to mother their children and they had hope for the future, despite the challenges. Mental health and homelessness, in particular, challenged their self-determination. Breastfeeding rates were low, and given the clear benefits, women should be strongly encouraged to do so and should be integrated into all Australian guidelines. Nurse-led models of care have the potential for improved access to HCV treatment.

Meta-theme 2: Trauma and sub-themes IPV and OOHC and relational issues

> 'I lost him in February, and then…I had a baby in September, and they took him from birth too…Well, I ran from the hospital'

Women interviewed for this study experienced multiple types of trauma, including IPV and child removal. Consequently, these traumas had profound impacts on the way the women perceived the world around them. Women felt let down and abandoned by health and social care providers and DCJ workers which is contradictory to the notion of these women being 'hard to reach'; they wanted care, just in the right way. This section focuses on impacts of IPV and OOHC. Contraception is discussed in this section and it is hypothesised that trauma is linked to low contraceptive rates and a repeat pregnancy, or replacement baby. The role of professional relationships are discussed.

Intimate Partner Violence

Intimate Partner Violence is a global public health issue and a serious social and economic burden to society (Mitchell, 2011, WHO, 2022). It is associated with SUD, injury, behavioural and emotional disturbances for children who witness violence and child removal into care (WHO, 2022). The response to IPV in Australia consists of ambitious targets, goals and policies, and a collaborative approach between the states and territories. These include awareness-raising, shifting cultural beliefs and recognising and responding to violence quickly so that women can rebuild their lives and be free from violence (COAG, 2020). This aligns with the United Nations sustainable development goal, 5, target 5.2, which aims to end all violence against women and the exploitation of women and girls (WHO, 2022). In 2020-2021, Australia pledged $538.1 million in funding over four years to prevent and respond to IPV (NCOSS, 2021). However, this has met criticism over a lack of short-term funding, and a limited funding for frontline services, long waiting lists, and a paucity of case management services (NCOSS, 2021).

The number of women experiencing IPV in this study was extremely high, where 12 of the 13 divulged violence. These rates appear to be even higher than other studies of women with SUDs. A Canadian study found rates of IPV in cohorts of women with SUDs were 56% (Cormier et al., 2004). Two Australian studies identified IPV rates of 17% of 54 pregnant women (Tsantefski et al., 2014) and Taplin and Mattick (2013) found that 18% of 171 mothers on an OAT program 171 women had an AVO taken out against their partner within six months of interview. While these rates are lower than in this current study, the rates are high across all studies and more research is required to understand the breadth of the issue.

The devastating effect that IPV had on pregnant and parenting included a cascade of physical trauma, psychosocial trauma, escalating drug use, and issues related to power and control (WHO, 2013). These issues can lead to further consequences such injury, fear of authorities due to the risk of child protection notifications, BBVIs, overdose and death. Furthermore, IPV can contribute to a lack of sexual and reproductive health control leading to none, or ineffective contraception (WHO, 2013). This could partly explain the absence of contraception for women in this study.

Entrenched violence, as identified by DCJ workers, was challenging to address and they sounded perplexed and defeated on the issue. Workers described challenges in identifying and responding to IPV and were particularly challenged when a woman chose to stay within a violent relationship. DCJ workers described mothers as having a difficult choice; to either stay with their partner, or have their children removed. There were no compromises and this created tension for women who wanted help for their partner's violence, but little was available.

The lack of confidence of health care and DCJ workers to deal with violence is problematic. This may be due to the siloed nature of health and government systems (Humphreys et al., 2021) that are not set up to address multiple complexities such as IPV, mental health and SUDs simultaneously. These issues are highly correlated and should be addressed together (Mason and O'Rinn, 2014). Moreover, current systems such as OAT services are not historically set up for women, and women may find it hard to access treatment alone, due to the presence of the perpetrator (García-Moreno et al., 2015).

Women only services, such as residential rehabilitation, do provide domestic violence programs and this was offered at least in eight of the services reviewed. The usefulness of these programs was questioned by both women and health care providers who noted the programs were not always valued or effective, but more a tick-a-box exercise to satisfy the requirements from DCJ. Interviewed women who had previously completed these programs complained as they found them repetitive. This was also identified in the literature review where women felt that some treatments were burdensome (Kuo et al., 2013), reducing acceptability of care (Levesque et al., 2013). Shared decision-making regarding treatment choices should be practiced to allow for greater autonomy; this can lead to greater willingness to engage in care (Friedrichs et al., 2016).

Furthermore, the utility of domestic violence programs in the perinatal period is unclear. A recent Cochrane review found so few high quality research studies on the topic that it was difficult to ascertain whether programs were helpful. Of ten randomised control trials comprising 3417 women, there was limited evidence for reducing episodes of violence (physical, sexual, and/or psychological) and preventing violence during and up to one year after pregnancy. This review recommended that high-quality studies are required that should include the voices of women to understand their preferences for care (Jahanfar et al., 2014).

The identification of violence in the first place is essential. One practice in NSW designed to capture the occurrence of IPV in pregnancy is the Domestic Violence Screening Tool (DVST) (NSW Health, 2006a), which should occur during antenatal assessments and should be undertaken by child and family health nurse postnatally. This tool can be helpful in the identification of violence but relies on effective referral pathways and trained staff who can appropriately respond. Limitations of the tool include not being able to screen due to the presence of a male partner, a lack of confidence from staff, and other staffing issues such as having enough time (O'Doherty et al., 2015). Some professionals regarded the tool as a 'tick-a-box exercise', that does not elicit the true extent of the violence. However, screening is better than not screening, but more research is needed on the effectiveness of screening (O'Doherty et al., 2015). The DVST must be added to the RANZCOG guidelines, as many women seek GP care throughout their pregnancy.

This current study found discrepancies between the identification of violence between the NSW Health DVST and the qualitative interviews, with more women divulging IPV during the qualitative interviews (9/13, vs 12/13). These findings indicate that more information is acquired when a conversation is undertaken instead of only using the tool. Also, the DVST form is designed to screen recent IPV (the previous 12 months). Unless the health professional has a good rapport with a woman, it may not trigger a conversation around past violence and trauma associated with IPV.

Reforms in NSW to respond to violence include Safer Pathways, which began in 2014, have been beneficial in identifying serious violence and includes a suite of actions including interagency safety meetings, and tools to identify the level of threat and refer appropriately (NSW Govt, 2019).

Evaluations of Safer Pathways found the program provided a systematic, state-wide response to IPV in NSW, supported by police, other government agencies and NGOs (NSW Govt, 2019). However, it recognised that Aboriginal people warrant particular attention due to high rates of IPV but those with SUDs were not, indicating that these women are missing from the picture (Hamilton, 2017).

Furthermore, this program relies on people coming forward, either to an emergency department (ED) or police and a skilled workforce can effectively identify and respond appropriately. However, a recent study from NSW found staff in EDs feel ill-equipped to deal with IPV, and some staff were not aware that the DV screening tool exists (Dawson et al., 2019).

More novel programs to address IPV should be examined. One such model is the STACY project (Staying Together Addressing ComplexitY). This model recognised the intersection of IPV, SUD and mental health and highlights the need to support each family member in their own right. This is done through targeted interventions that holds perpetrators accountable for their abuse, while ensuring the safety and wellbeing of women and children through partnering with the non-offending parent (usually the mother). This approaches challenges entrenched practices that render fathers who use violence invisible, and judge mothers through as a 'failure to protect' (Humphreys et al., 2021)

Out of home care, grief and loss

A dearth of literature provides information on women experiencing involuntary child removal (Marsh et al., 2019). When a mother loses a child to stillbirth, miscarriage or even adoption, society sympathises with the woman, allowing her to grieve (Nichols et al., 2021b). Yet, if a mother loses a child to the child protection system, it is 'her fault' and she is doubly stigmatised by society as a morally deviant mother who cannot care for her child, and as a drug user (Nichols et al., 2021b). This can lead to feelings of guilt, isolation and stigma (Broadhurst and Mason, 2017), and anger towards child protection services and can impact health care engagement in subsequent pregnancies (Lewis, 2006). Anger can lead to, disengagement from care, escalating drug use (Broadhurst and Mason, 2017, Broadhurst and Mason, 2019), a return to IPV and a repeated pregnancy (Wise, 2020). This is known as collateral damage of child removal (Broadhurst and Mason, 2017). Part of this vicious cycle must be interrupted (Wise, 2020), to prevent further collateral damage, such as addressing the substance use or grief.

This study captured important data from a hidden population of women who almost all (11/13) had children removed into OOHC. These findings contribute to the emerging body of work in Australia and Internationally that explores experiences from women's perspectives (Broadhurst and Mason, 2019, Hinton, 2018, Ross et al., 2017, Broadhurst and Mason, 2017, Broadhurst et al., 2015). Listening to the stories of women in this PhD study who had children removed was difficult. Their accounts of how child removal took place revealed a picture of immense pain, grief and loss. It is important to note, at times, women described moments of gratitude when the removal took place more compassionately and kindly, demonstrating the importance of empathetic care (Kramlich and Kronk, 2015).

Programs and support services in NSW for women experiencing child removal, include primary health services, mental health, drug and alcohol treatment services, legal services, and non-government support services. Critically, this study found that few women access services at this time and 'go underground' as they are caught in a cycle of grief. Therefore, care should be delivered at the time of removal which has the potential to mitigate consequences of collateral damage (Broadhurst and Mason, 2017, Broadhurst and Mason, 2019). Care should be provided as long as is required including grief counselling and support to manage their emotions, (Memarnia et al., 2015, Broadhurst et al., 2015). A model that promotes continuity of care (Marsh et al., 2019) within a trauma-informed model is best suited for women at this time as this has been demonstrated to decrease substance use, depressive and trauma symptoms (Covington et al., 2008).

Programs to support women with children in OOHC in Australia are sparse. One service in the Hunter region in NSW trialled a peer support program for mothers with children in OOHC. This program holds some promise, but further work is required. This program, while still in its infancy has been valued by parents, peers and by the broad range of agencies involved (Cocks et al., 2021). However, it is underfunded, and it became clear that the peers, as well as the parents needed a lot of support, given the trauma background by both cohorts. Unfortunately, this program has been interrupted by the Covid-19 pandemic, but some limited work in this area is continuing (Cocks et al., 2021).

This study found child removal was distressing for the workforce involved. In particular, child protection staff face the brunt of this distress and can lead to high staff turnover, stress, compassion fatigue and vicarious trauma (Russ et al., 2009, Molnar et al., 2020, Ashley-Binge and Cousins, 2020). If unmanaged, this distress can be detrimental to staff and the families they are working with in the long term. Reforms in Australia's child protection industry include moving from deficit to strengths and resilience-based models to improve outcomes for families, better support staff, and reduce attrition (Russ et al., 2009).

Reflective practice and supervision for DCJ workers are recommended and vital to maintaining a strong child protection workforce (Russ et al., 2009, Hunt et al., 2016). However, from the DCJ workers' perspectives, this happened haphazardly or not at all. Some sought external supervision in their own time, with their own money, demonstrating an inconsistent approach to care for these workers which can impact families they are providing care for. A robust child protection system requires a strong workforce (Russ et al., 2022)

This study found that some child protection workers experienced challenges working with Aboriginal families due to the high levels of trauma in women, their families and communities. These challenges are described in the literature and s can lead to poor outcomes for Aboriginal women (Menzies and Grace, 2022). As a result, there is a need for high-quality training in entry-level and ongoing professional development in trauma-informed care practice for DCJ workers within a cultural competence framework (Herring et al., 2013). Aboriginal liaison officers who work at DCJ can help create a culture and environment that is more acceptable to Aboriginal populations, but DCJ workers found them in high demand and not always available due to competing priorities.

Contraception

None of the eligible ten post-partum women in this study were on contraception. Low contraceptive uptake in women with SUDs is consistent with the literature (Black et al., 2012a, Terplan et al., 2015). Unmet need for contraception must be addressed as this can lead to a repeat pregnancy or a 'replacement baby' (Broadhurst et al., 2015, Hinton, 2018). Benefits of providing contraception for vulnerable women with SUDs include allowing time to rehabilitate, enter SUD treatment, parent their current children, and deal with grief if their child was removed (Broadhurst et al., 2015). In addition, the WHO recommends there should be two years between children as this is optimal for maternal and infant health (WHO, 2007).

Interviewed health care workers explained women might not have easy access to contraceptive care. Therefore, integrating SRH care such as long-acting reversible contraception (LARC) into drug treatment settings may reduce barriers and increase uptake. Implanon which is a progesterone implant is the ideal option as it lasts three years, it is 99.95% effective and is relatively simple to insert (Fischer, 2008). The few programs that provide this service in SUDs treatment services have yielded mixed results. Barriers to care such as stigma, competing priorities, structural barriers, lack of knowledge on SRH services and substance use, fear of child protection notifications and cost and expertise of staff to deliver SRH care may impact service uptake (Black and Day, 2016, MacAfee et al., 2020).

One measure to overcome these barriers is a nurse-led model of care. Access to contraception can be improved by upskilling registered nurses, in the provision of LARC (Botfield et al., 2020). Training includes online learning, simulated practice, and supervised clinical training with a competency assessment (Botfield et al., 2021). Internationally, nurse provision of LARC is widely practiced such as in the UK and Sweden (Botfield et al., 2021). Unfortunately, there no provision for nurses to provide services or claim for LARC procedures through the MBS in Australia meaning that there would be no payment from the government for this service in the public sector (Botfield et al., 2021).

The provision of LARC by nurses however is cost effective. Botfield et al. (2020) found that when they reviewed the uptake of LARC, in-line with comparable countries, the value of avoided abortions and miscarriages would be $20 million over five years. In Australia, if 20% of women who switch to a LARC, are provided with services by a nurse (compared to a GP), there would be a government saving of $2.7 million (Botfield et al., 2020), indicating that this is a cost-effective option. Settings that provide nurse-led models of care have been demonstrated to be accessible and acceptable in populations of people with SUDs (Fedele, 2020, Papaluca et al., 2019). The provision of LARC in PHC settings is also a viable option. Women also need to be educated about their menstrual cycle and pregnancy risk. Irregular menstrual cycles secondary to substance use (Schmittner et al., 2005) may lead women to believe they cannot fall pregnant as they are not mensurating regularly.

One model of SRH care, the Pause Program, involves women taking a break from pregnancy and using contraception for 18 months. This program from the UK, aims to provide mothers with children in OOHC the time they need to heal and address their trauma (Pause, 2020). Children are placed at the centre of care, and women are encouraged to take responsibility for their actions, to focus on their and their children's needs and include relationship building and maintaining contact (Pause, 2020). While the program is subject to ongoing evaluations, 125 women have completed the program. This program has reduced unintended pregnancies in the 18-month interventional period, ultimately reducing the number of children entering care (Boddy et al., 2020).

No such model of care provision exists in Australia, however 'Pause' could be integrated into care provision. Furthermore, Pause is not incentivised, such as the USA program, Project Prevention, where mothers were paid $300 cash to access contraception (Lucke and Hall, 2012) and so may be more acceptable in the Australian context, as cash incentives are viewed as ethically controversial (Won et al., 2017).

Ethically, health professionals, must consider the woman's interest in contraception at the point of care and respect her self-determination and not speculate about possible future risks (Wale and Rowlands, 2021). Women must have full capacity to make informed choices about their sexual and reproductive health care (Broadhurst et al., 2015), and this can be more difficult to ensure in women with SUDs. These women may find it more difficult to exercise their reproductive rights than other cohorts of women due to being disempowered, IPV, substance misuse, and reproductive coercion (Broadhurst et al., 2015). For these women, a proactive approach to SRH care including contraception must be part of holistic care and if she does fall pregnant, as health care workers we must ensure equitable access to health care (Broadhurst et al., 2015).

Professional relationships and care providers
An interesting finding in this study was that women's relationships with health and social care and DCJ workers were key to women's outcomes. Women spoke positively of relationships built on trust and respect and when their concerns were heard. This suggests that empathy and therapeutic alliance can significantly influence addiction treatment outcomes (Miller and Moyers, 2015). Relationships between women and their key workers are rarely described in the literature as they are not treatments as such. However, the treatments and interventions that women are provided with exist in a contextual and a relational setting, and the 'soft-skills' (Miller and Moyers, 2015) alongside the provision of health care are valued by women. Women noticed when care was delivered sensitively, and they identified situations when staff were burnt out, and lacked enthusiasm and empathy. Health care workers must strive to build positive relationships with their clients as this is critical to engagement with vulnerable women. Therapeutic communication as a skill set needs to be valued, and the workforce should be adequately skilled (Bartlett et al., 2013).

Support provided to women in a way that respected their values and preferences for care was appreciated by the women. The women described a sense of abandonment when support was withdrawn, such as being discharged from the hospital, DCJ care, or when a child was removed into OOHC. Some women were angry and felt betrayed. Lack of ongoing support for women is also highlighted as an issue in the literature (Taplin et al., 2015, Coupland et al., 2021) and will be further discussed in Meta-theme 4. There appears to be very little to nothing in contemporary literature describing this sense of abandonment or betrayal. This may stem from trauma histories and poor attachment to primary caregivers as children, leading to disorganised attachment styles as adults

(Holmes, 2014). Women in these situations are most likely stressed, leading to maladaptive coping mechanisms. They may not perceive the need to reach out or know how to access further care at this difficult time (Sinha, 2008). A sense of abandonment also supports the idea of women as foetal containers (Ettorre, 2015) where a mother's rights are overridden by others such as child protection authorities and that the mother is no longer needed.

Findings from this meta-theme identified high rates of IPV and trauma from child removal. This trauma meant that some women had a repeat pregnancy to replace a removed child. Nurse-led and midwifery-led models of care can assist women to become empowered regarding their SRH so women can access timely and appropriate care. This meta-theme found that relational aspects to care were very important and gaps in services regarding follow up care for women exist.

Meta-theme 3: Power, surveillance and stigma

> 'Everyone like, pulling strings for you. Like a puppet...I don't even get to pee by myself. I have to pee on cue'

This section will discuss the role of power, surveillance, and stigma on women interviewed for this study. The power within health and social care environments played a significant role in how women felt and interacted with care, which impacted their health-seeking behaviours and, consequently, health outcomes. Recognising power imbalances and working to seek to shift this imbalance is central to the tenet of feminism and, therefore, crucial to this research (Dunkerley, 2017). Furthermore, stigma, is a resource that can be used in society to exert power over people. Hence power and stigma are inextricably linked (Link and Phelan, 2014).

Power

The women's lack of power and autonomy over their lives and their children left them angry, frustrated, and confused. This included situations that directly affected them, such as being reported to child protection or when they were not informed that their children were removed. Women wished they were afforded information pertinent to their futures, but it may be that care providers deem providing this information to women unsafe. In the context of very high rates of IPV, care providers may fear retribution for the women or children, including escalation of violence or threats of harm (Felson et al., 2002, Voce and Boxall, 2018). A further consequence identified by DCJ workers is a concern women may leave from the hospital with their baby on their own accord. Open, honest and timely conversations should be occurring with women, and transparency is part of child protection practice in NSW (DCJ, 2021a).

Women explicitly used the term 'power' to describe imbalances in interactions with staff, demonstrating that they were acutely aware of the dynamics. These power dynamics were recognised and acknowledged by health and social care providers and the DCJ workers as an issue that pervades their practice. However, one DCJ worker described these power dynamics as an inherent part of care provision.

Definitions of power are 'the capacity of some persons to produce intended and foreseen effects on others' (Wrong, 2017p.2) and the provision of one person or a group of people who have an ability to exert control over others' lives (Foucault, 1982). For example, at the macro level, governments can exercise control or choice at the micro (individual and group) level (Laverack, 2004). Sometimes we willingly accept this macro-level ability, such as in legislation to prevent or punish crimes against people (Laverack, 2004). Other times we do not. One contemporary example is Covid-19 vaccine mandates for health workers, where the majority of people accept this level of power at the macro level, but a minority have risen from the fringes to form anti-vaccination groups to protest against the government as they feel it is a breach of human rights (Bing, 2022).

The discourse around power is highly relevant to conversations around health and social care provision where themes of power, dominance, and hierarchy exist (O'Shea et al., 2019). Power imbalances in health care are pervasive, especially as medical doctors hold power through knowledge, expertise, and prestige. In contrast, patients or health care consumers traditionally hold less power (Foucault, 2003). These power imbalances extend to other environments such as through social care providers who decide whether a mother gets to keep her child or not (Bunton and Petersen, 2002).

Positively, more recently, the patient/public have become better informed about illnesses and treatments and have become self-advocates for their health care. This has the potential to narrow the power disparity. Unfortunately, this does not apply to all groups where women, low socioeconomic groups and other vulnerable groups may lack the resources to question decisions or challenge prescribed care (Foucault, 2003). Women throughout history have been disempowered and viewed as subordinate, placing women at greater risk of illness and diseases such as HIV (Wingood and DiClemente, 2000) and HCV (Fraser et al., 2014).

The inclusion of consumers and peers regarding support and decision making in health care is increasing. Within the area of addiction services this model shows much promise and can lead to better engagement in treatment, greater acceptability of care and has the potential to shift power dynamics. Further research is needed to further expand on this important line of research (Bryant et al., 2021, Tracy and Wallace, 2016).

Surveillance and the burden of proof

Alongside the notion of power were themes of surveillance and the burden of proof were identified in this research. Women had to prove to the 'authorities' that they could be good mothers. Women who described these scenarios did so with an element of acceptance. One woman said having to provide proof was 'fair enough'. This complacency and acceptance of highly unusual situations such as having to prove your ability to mother, is an outcome of policy decisions at the macro level, designed to control vulnerable groups (Laverack, 2004). An example is urine drug screening which, as mentioned in the guideline review, has limited utility, yet this study found, some women were asked to undertake this screening practice and while women agreed, they did so as they had no choice.

Women wanted support from their DCJ and health care workers but did not want to be monitored and surveyed. But because society views mothers with SUDs as morally deviant (Nichols et al., 2021b), their mothering is observed and critiqued at every step, from pregnancy to birth, and beyond. In exchange for giving up their power, women expected consistency, fairness and transparency from care providers. Women were especially frustrated when DCJ workers kept 'changing the gaol posts'; they had held up their end of the bargain, and so why couldn't they. 'Changing the goal posts' left women confused. One woman was informed that she would be reunified with her children if she completed rehabilitation. This reunification did not occur, and she was instructed to meet further criteria. The decision to 'move the goal posts' angered women and health care workers who corroborated these stories. Health care workers were perplexed at decisions made by DCJ at times that did not always make sense.

Forming positive relationships between women and DCJ workers is inherently tricky and laden with power dynamics, especially for women who previously had had a child removed. Therefore, it is critical that these power dynamics are shifted, enabling women to be central participants in their own care, instead of silent partners. Providing care that respects principles of autonomy, the values of individuals, and involving people in their care decisions are important determinants for empowerment (Sharma et al., 2015). Examples of ways this shift could include involving women in selecting service providers and being responsive to their input about needed services. Power-sharing (Dunkerley, 2017), through the provision of options for women, was identified as necessary in the literature review. Meeting the needs of mothers does not have to be at the expense of the children,

and it also says to women that they matter too, and deserve to have their needs addressed
(Dunkerley, 2017).

Stigma

Stigma affects an individual's emotional, mental, and physical health and is related to poor
outcomes, such as failure to access treatment, disempowerment, reduced self-efficacy, decreased
quality of life and acceptability of health care (Yang et al., 2017, Cheng et al., 2019, Levesque et al.,
2013). People with a SUD are often viewed as unpredictable, dangerous, and morally responsible for
their condition which perpetuates the stigma even further (Yang et al., 2017). The stigma of mothers
with SUDs is so profound that some women evade health care in the first place, and when they do
present for care, they are met with attitudes linked to the stereotypes associated with drug use
(Brener et al., 2019, Olsen et al., 2012).

Stigma was a prominent finding throughout this current study, and it was mentioned in 11 of the 20
studies in the literature review. While these findings are well known, it must be emphasised that
impacts of stigma from health care staff can have long lasting negative effects that may not be
remedied over time. This includes disengagement from care at critical time points and low levels of
breastfeeding. This is essential information for health care providers to be made aware of as this can
provide an opportunity to reflect on their stereotypes.

One interesting finding was the stigma felt by health and social care providers. They described being
stigmatised because of working with stigmatised individuals (Ahmedani, 2011). This is known as
associated stigma and this can directly affect patient care (Ahmedani, 2011), lead to professional
identity issues, a lack of belonging in the workplace and high staff turnover and burnout (Eaton et
al., 2015, Corrigan et al., 2011). This demonstrates that more efforts are required to increase
resilience and reduce workforce stigma in the sector, protect the workers and, most importantly, the
vulnerable women they work with (Kulesza et al., 2017).

Another interesting impact of associated stigma elicited in interviews was that stigma impacted
funding for the sector. Minimal research exists in this area, but Yang et al. (2017) stated that this
stigma might explain why few individuals receive the SUD services they need. They also recommend
that widespread public education about the benefits of SUD treatment is required.

According to the stigma reduction theory, core elements for reducing stigma include education,
contact, and protest (Corrigan and Penn, 1999). In the context of SUDs, education provides

information about addiction and seeks to dispel associated myths; contact includes interactions with people with SUDs (such as those with lived experience); and protest is where one is encouraged to speak out against prejudices and discriminatory acts towards people with a SUD (Corrigan et al., 2001). Unfortunately and of note, stigma reduction is not integrated into health care delivery, nor is it evaluated or regularly integrated into pre-service and in-service training of health care workers (Nyblade et al., 2019). Furthermore, health care workers may be unaware of how stigma affects people and may not be cognizant of the stigmatising effects of their actions. Health workers may also be unaware how stigma influences health facilities' policies or structures affect clients (Nyblade et al., 2019). Therefore, tackling stigma requires a multileveled approach across the spectrum of the socioecological model, that addressed stigma from an individual through to a policy level.

This meta-theme reveals that women are interacting with a paternalistic healthcare, social welfare and child protection system that is both disempowering and punitive. Women wanted help and they understood that the role of child protection is to oversee their care and their interactions with their children. However, women wanted transparency and to be equal partners in their care. This meta-theme also revealed that stigma is rife in health care settings affecting staff and client outcomes. A multileveled approach to tackle stigma is required.

Meta-theme 4: Systemic issues

'They're just setting me up to fail'

Lack of timely treatment, a stable home, and follow up care were issues highlighted by all cohorts interviewed for this study. These issues left women confounded and this contributed to escalating drug use, lack of trust in systems and affected outcomes regarding child protection and permanency planning. This section will discuss the systemic issues that had profound impacts on women's lives and limitations and gaps in care

Treatment access

Many people interviewed for this study described long waiting lists for treatment, including residential rehabilitation, methadone, and one woman waited for specialist antenatal care. Waiting lists for treatment were similarly identified in the situational analysis, and the literature review. Problematically, it is estimated that fewer than half of those seeking AOD treatment can access it (Ritter and Stoove, 2016). The lack of timely treatment access has serious consequences, including homelessness, substance use, anxiety, and disrupted mother-infant attachment as mothers waited for treatment while their baby was in OOHC.

The lack of treatment places for women is out of step with Australia's harm reduction approach to SUDs (Ritter et al., 2014) and is also a challenge in other similar high income countries (Kohn et al., 2004). The lack of treatment places is a problematic as it denies beneficial treatment for pregnant women and women with children (Jones et al., 2006, Niccols et al., 2012, Suchman et al., 2006, Doab et al., 2015). Furthermore, and as outlined in the background of this study, SUD treatment is a good return on investment. Promisingly, in the 2016-17 Budget, the NSW Government announced $197 million for drug and alcohol services. This included $15 million for substance use in pregnancy support and $8 million to increase residential rehabilitation places for parents with children (NSW Health, 2017a). However, this funding has been criticised for not considering specialised needs of pregnant women and women with children, and children were not included in the costings. Nor did it account for the substantial amount of time clinical staff spend managing complex issues such as liaising with DCJ (NADA, 2019). Promise for more novel methods such as the use of nurse practitioners in the AOD setting includes increased access to services, reduced waiting times, improved quality of treatment. But expansion of the nurse practitioner role is required (Ling, 2009).

Appropriate housing
A lack of appropriate housing impacted women's stability, and safety and influenced child protection worker's decisions regarding permanency planning. Social housing in Australia is at a crisis point and there is a shrinking social housing market (Pawson et al., 2019), with waiting lists for housing, up to ten years (AIHW, 2021b). While there are priority groups for social housing, such as those who are homeless or at immediate risk of homelessness, women and children are not a priority group (AIHW, 2021b). Women had to take whatever home they were allocated, even if it did not meet their needs. For example, the placement of women in areas with high levels of marginalisation and drug dealers tempted women with low incomes to make money through drug dealing. Some women saw using drugs as a way to connect socially and make extra income.

There are few options for many women with SUDs to leave social housing, especially in Australia, where there is a lack of affordable and secure housing options available to low-income earners. Women who have the resources leave others behind to remain in marginalised neighbourhoods and in social housing that is associated with crime, anti-social behaviours and welfare dependency (AHURI, 2019). This situation makes it easy to understand why the women in this study felt that they are set up to fail.

COVID-19 has also impacted housing availability. Combined with the already high numbers of women fleeing IPV, more must be done to address the housing shortage so that pregnant women can access permanent housing and obtain stability early in their pregnancy. This will improve outcomes for both mother and child (Murray et al., 2018).

A lack of timely treatment access and appropriate housing are incompatible with the child protection policy that aims to plan for permanency within two years of child removal (DCJ, 2021a), if reunification is not possible. This means that circumstances beyond a woman's control have a real potential to make restoration plans challenging to achieve.

Gaps in policy and care

This research identified three key areas that need to be addressed: a rigorous review and evaluation of Perinatal Family Conferencing (PFC), more targeted care in early childhood and support for women with children OOHC.

Reforms in NSW include PFC and prenatal reporting, which allows a child protection notification to be made whilst the mother is still pregnant (Taplin et al., 2015). Perinatal family conferencing utilises an interagency strength-based approach model to plan and implement support for pregnant women (Taplin et al., 2015). Findings from this current study found health and social care workers valued PFC overall and appreciated its interagency approach. This is similar to findings to a study by (Coupland et al., 2021) where they explored service providers' perceptions of key components of a model of care for a substance use in parenting services program in Sydney, NSW. They also identified benefits of PFC that included empowering women and identifying strengths. However, in this PhD study, differing approaches and philosophies between health and social care providers and DCJ created tension. For example, midwives provide women-centred care, whereas DCJ provide child-centred care. Midwives felt frustrated that DCJ had the final say, especially when they had a differing view. While there is support for the PFC program, it has not been rigorously reviewed. This lack of a review does not mean that the program is not beneficial. Evidence of effectiveness and the inclusion of women's voices and how they perceive care is required to improve the quality and outcomes of these programs.

Health care workers and DCJ identified gaps in care for women and their children who were discharged from DCJ care. With few ongoing supports, risk of IPV and unsuitable housing, this set women up to fail. Programs designed to assist vulnerable families, such as Sustaining Families NSW do not appear to meet the needs of women interviewed for this study. Sustaining Families NSW is a home visiting model of care for vulnerable families experiencing social and economic disadvantage and associated mental health and wellbeing impacts. This program is designed to give children the best start in life and is led by nurses, ideally commencing during pregnancy until the child's second birthday (Turnbull and Osborn, 2012). Unfortunately, the program misses extremely vulnerable families who are identified as unsuited to this program. There is insufficient evidence to recommend home visits for women with SUDs, indicating a gap in care provision for these vulnerable communities of women and children (Turnbull and Osborn, 2012).

One suitable program is Brighter Futures which provides intense support to vulnerable families up until the child is nine years of age (NSW Govt, 2021). This program has positive gains regarding child protection notifications and entry into care for some families. However, an evaluation of the program found that the families had multiple and complex issues that were difficult to address, and suggested that an integrated case management model involving better collaboration between multiple government and NGO service providers would be beneficial (Social Policy Research Centre, 2010). It is unknown if women in this current study were referred to this program. Several health care workers observed very little support for mothers with children aged from 18 months until the child starts school. The outcome of minimal support for these families results in them 'falling through all the cracks' and out of sight, until a crisis ensues.

An alternative intervention for Australia for parents with SUD who have children in OOHC, a trial status in Victoria, is the Family Drug Treatment Court (FDTC). Unlike an ordinary court, the FDTC is underpinned by a theory known as therapeutic jurisprudence (Winick, 2002) that treats parents within the court. This program is unique as it balances the parental needs alongside a child's right to timely permanency (Harwin et al., 2019). The program provides intensive case coordination and holistic intervention to address SUDs and aims to achieve safe and sustainable family reunification of parents and their children. Evaluations of FDTCs in the USA and Australia have found better reunification rates, attributed mainly to success in addressing parental substance misuse than standard treatment models or court (Worcel et al., 2008, De Bortoli et al., 2018, Dakof et al., 2010). Criticisms of FDTC are that it focuses largely on reunification and cessation of drug use without adequate attention to mental health, domestic violence, and even less on entry into employment or retraining and issues associated with poverty (Harwin et al., 2019). Nevertheless, its approach has been lauded as ground-breaking within an area with so few novel approaches and its utility in Australia should be further explored.

Findings in this meta-theme found that structural barriers make it difficult for women to achieve positive outcomes because of issues beyond their control. A lack of timely treatment entry and suitable housing profoundly impacts women and their children's lives and highlights that women are set up to fail. Gaps in care provision and novel programs mean that women miss out on essential care that has the potential to improve outcomes. Research and programs such as the FDTC could be expanded and trialled in the NSW context.

Summary

This study sought to understand the needs and experiences of pregnant women and new mothers with a history of injecting drug use. Understanding their needs, experiences and preferences for care enables health care and policymakers to work towards a model of care that meets their needs. Overall, this study found multiple health and psychosocial needs, including addiction, mental health disorders, hepatitis C and SRH needs. Women were highly traumatised and experienced high levels of IPV and many had a child in OOHC.

Health, social care and DCJ workers interviewed for this study were highly skilled and passionate professionals who wanted the best outcomes for their clients and to make a difference. However, their efforts were hampered by stigma at a service level, and they were stigmatised for the work they do; and some staff believed that stigma at a broader level impacted funding for their services. In addition, efforts to provide care were difficult due to fragmented care systems, structural barriers and working with women experiencing trauma, substance use, mental health disorders and violence. At times, care providers and DCJ workers were ill equipped to address their clients' multiple needs and were perplexed when women did not access care, or stayed in violent relationships. In particular, DCJ workers found their jobs stressful, and some were traumatised due to the nature of their work and this impacted care provision. Supervision models to support DCJ staff were inconsistent.

Structural barriers for women meant they faced homelessness or housing that did not meet their needs, and at times they had to wait for treatment access. This lack of suitable and timely access to care frustrated health, social care and DCJ workers. They described injustices in the systems and structural barriers that impacted women's outcomes even further as some women continued to use substances and were homeless, all the while, their babies were bonding with OOHC providers, and a chance of reunification moved further into the distance.

Despite support from care providers, women experienced enormous challenges at every level. However, they had a firm belief in their ability to parent. The women had hopes and dreams to be a 'good' mother. They demonstrated enormous strength and resilience under extremely difficult circumstances as they navigated their way through models of care that were stigmatising, scrutinising and surveyed their every move. This left women powerless at times and many accepted this as normal practice. This lack of power over many aspects of their lives may have provided a pathway for women to seek control over other areas of their lives such as contraception, choosing to fall pregnant and choice of partner. Decisions that were not always viewed favourably by care providers and DCJ workers.

Therapeutic communication should drive interactions between health, social care providers and DCJ. This approach ensures that care is empathetic and respectful and can positively impact difficult conversations that care providers need to have with women regarding child protection matters. Not all women in his study were in a position to have their babies and children remain in their care at the time of interview. However, this should not be the end point of care but a part of women's journey. Care needs to extend beyond child removal, not just because these women may have a repeated pregnancy, but because they deserve care like any other person with a chronic disease or illness.

Strengths and limitations

This study is unique to the Australian landscape. It has given women who were either pregnant, or parenting, and are current injecting drug users a platform to voice their needs and experiences. This study included both women with and without custody of their children and differs from other Australian studies in the field, such as those by Hinton (2018), Ross et al. (2017) who specifically examine the experiences of mothers who have their children removed into OOHC.

This research was strengthened by the inclusion of multiple perspectives (Yin, 2014) from women, health care and social care providers and DCJ workers. Multiple perspectives are essential for verifying and understanding any areas of cognitive dissonance and obtaining a broad view of the situation. Furthermore, while there were many socio-demographical similarities amongst the recruited women, they came from a range of cultural backgrounds. Five women identified as Aboriginal, two women identified as Asian and one woman as Persian and the remaining five identified as Anglo-Saxon demonstrating diversity in perspectives. Hearing the voices of women with diverse backgrounds is essential to understand if there are different cultural needs (EMCDDA, 2017).

The use of validated screening tools enhanced the reliability of the study (Plano Clark and Ivankova, 2016), however the AGREE II tool, which was used to assess the clinical guidelines, can result in subjective responses, and some argue that it is problematic as the scores are all equal, with no weighting (Brosseau et al., 2014, Greenfield et al., 2004).

This study has some limitations related to the study design and sampling bias. Case study and mixed methods research have been criticised as not generalisable, subjective, and only suited to pilot studies (Flyvbjerg, 2006). On the contrary, Flyvbjerg (2006) argues that case studies contribute to understanding phenomena and can uncover a greater depth of knowledge than traditional study types with larger sample sizes. This study aimed to reduce bias that are inherent within mixed methods study design by ensuring that reliability and rigour were addressed. This is described in the methods section. This also included strict protocols to be enacted if required, of which was not needed.

All participants were recruited from a convenience sample. Convenience sampling can contribute to bias as the sample is not representative. This can lead to sampling bias and cannot be extrapolated to other populations (Etikan et al., 2016, Sousa et al., 2004). Eleven of the 13 women recruited resided in rehabilitation settings at the time, so there is limited knowledge of the needs of women living in the community. Efforts were made to recruit women from the community, although this was difficult due to low referral rates and difficulties in reaching women when contact attempts were made. In addition, this study aimed to interview all women over multiple time points; however, many women were lost to follow up and were only interviewed once, which can be typical of cohorts of people with SUDs (Horyniak et al., 2013, Mousavian et al., 2021). All health and social care providers and DCJ workers who were approached or referred to the study agreed to and participated, which demonstrates a willingness to contribute knowledge to the issues that women who are pregnant or new mothers with SUDs face.

This relatively small study focused on women's voices from inner-city Sydney. Women residing in other areas, such as suburban or regional areas, may have different or additional needs as resources in these areas are typically lacking (Barclay et al., 2018). There are some similarities between findings in this current study and other studies that explore similar issues (Broadhurst and Mason, 2017, Broadhurst and Mason, 2019, Broadhurst et al., 2015, Hinton, 2018, Ross et al., 2017). These similarities indicate that the findings may be relevant to other cohorts of pregnant women and mothers with SUDs. All women who took part in this research were accessing at least some service, such as OAT or residential drug treatment. Therefore, there may be different experiences for other populations of women who are even harder to reach.

Recommendations for Policy and Practice

'It takes a village to raise a child'

This final section provides recommendations for policy and practice to improve outcomes for pregnant women and new mothers with a history of injecting drug use. This study recommends a women-and infant-centred, strengths-based and trauma-informed model of care. Critically the model needs to support the development of the maternal infant relationship to increase the woman's ability to provide a secure base for her infant in times of distress, and the recognition by the woman of unsafe situations and appropriate interventions to manage these situations. Continuity of care model must be a part of care provision, underpinned by harm reduction, with a recognition of the impact of the social determinants of health on women's lives. These determinants include homelessness, poverty, racism, IPV and substance use. In addition, culturally appropriate care is essential when providing care to Aboriginal women. The provision of culturally safe and appropriate care must include programs that focus on self- determination of mothers, families, and communities, connection to culture and healing from intergenerational, historical, and lifetime trauma (Ritland et al., 2020).

Addressing SUDs in pregnant women and new mothers requires a coordinated effort involving tertiary substance use in pregnancy programs, community mental health services, domestic violence services, SUD treatment settings, primary health care settings, housing and DCJ. A one-stop-shop model of integrated primary health care is a recommended context where multiple issues can be addressed at once. This model must be supported by strength-based women-centred policies and guidelines otherwise change at the service or individual level may have limited impact.

Nurses and midwives in all NSW Health care settings have a responsibility to ensure people with drug and alcohol related issues experience person-centred, safe and high-quality interventions and care and this is embedded in NSW Health Policy (NSW Health, 2020). Further education and skills development of nurses and midwives working in the AOD sector is even more critical. This should be extended to all nurses and midwives working in child and family health, SRH and who work with women with SUDs. Lifelong learning must be supported by health managers and additional courses such as trauma informed care, infant and adult mental health nursing and AOD nursing would be beneficial. For example, specialist trained nurses in the field of AOD have found to be more confident to refer individuals with problematic AOD use for specialist assessment and treatment (Searby and Smyth, 2018). There are financial incentives in Australia for further tertiary study and nurses and midwives who hold post graduate qualifications, who are entitled to a continuing education allowance in addition to their salary (NSWNMA, 2021).

Implications for nursing practice.

Policies, guidelines and a one-stop-shop model of integrated primary health care that holistically meets the needs of women has the potential to break the cycle of adversity by addressing multiple layers of health and psychosocial issues. For example, relationship building with local health providers can facilitate a woman's access to OAT which can promote stability, and better health outcomes. This can be achieved through targeted outreach models that promote continuity of care.

One model of care that has the potential to make a difference is a sustained home visiting program (SHVP) specifically for women with SUDs. This program can be an expansion of existing substance use in pregnancy and parenting services (SUPPS) within Local Health Districts. The current SUPPS program is coordinated by a Clinical Nurse Consultant who works closely with midwives, doctors, social workers, treatment programs and DCJ workers. Additionally, a nurse led SVHP consisting of a highly skilled multidisciplinary team that supports a holistic approach to care should be employed. Clinicians such as midwives, SUPPS teams, family and childhood health nurses, mental health clinicians, addiction specialists as well as social workers should be part of this team. Multiple health and psychosocial needs can be addressed through this model including antenatal care, and rehabilitation.

Care provision should commence in early pregnancy irrespective of whether the women is accessing a residential rehabilitation program or if she is living in the community. This should include access to parenting programs, SUD treatment, a mental health clinician and domestic violence counselling if required. Social workers can link women into housing and liaise with other organisations such as DCJ. A small team of nurses should lead and coordinate the care which should continue at least until the child's first year or until the child begins school if required (NSW Govt, 2021). A small coordination team is recommended in order to build trust and bring consistency to these women's lives. In addition, this study found these professional relationships are important and valued. Consultations would not always have to be face to face but via telehealth and phone calls in between visits.

The SVHP model should be grounded in relevant empirically-based knowledge and should be underpinned by principles of empowerment (Zand et al., 2017, Stubbs and Achat, 2016). A highly skilled team must be able to recognise strengths within households as well as risks such as substance abuse, risk of child abuse and neglect, deteriorating mental health and the presence of violence, and balance the principles of harm reduction. Timely referrals as well as the need for child care are essential, and respite care for children while mothers build new knowledge may be necessary. For example, a mother may require extra support to parent in a more sensitive way, or it is identified that while a child is not an immediate risk of harm, they present with behavioural and learning difficulties that can have long lasting effects through childhood and into adulthood that require extra support, and at times developmentally appropriate interventions.

This SHVP must include care for women who have children removed into care. This should include immediate support and counselling at the time of child removal and an ongoing opportunity for women to address their issues such as substance abuse or mental health concerns. Access to timely SRH including contraception must be included in this model for all women. Programs such as 'Pause' should be trialled in the Australian context.

Rigorous testing compared to standard of care should be undertaken, preferably through an RCT. Outcome measures should include both maternal and child outcomes such as maternal health, child health, child development and school readiness, prevention of child abuse and neglect, increased parenting capacity, and maternal maintenance in SUD treatment.

Final recommendations:

1. All Australian guidelines used in practice should align with the WHO recommendations and include the provision of trauma-informed care, breastfeeding, sleeping practices, contraception, IPV and stigma, OAT and cultural considerations. In particular, the RANZCOG guidelines must include all of these missing components and this should be urgently addressed.

2. The provision of an appropriately educated workforce who are confident and competent in their practise (Marcellus, 2014) and can effectively and sensitively respond to women's needs. This education should include trauma-informed care models as well as stigma reduction both at the individual and the structural level for all staff involved in health care settings (Nyblade et al., 2019). This education should focus on deconstructing stereotypes and include understanding the impacts of stigma on women with SUDs

3. Intimate partner violence requires urgent attention. Women with SUDs should be included in NSW Health 2021-2026 Domestic Violence Strategy (MoH, 2012). Models that focus on better identification, better responses and continuity of care are needed. Projects such as the STACY could be expanded (Humphreys et al., 2021).

4. The trauma of working in the child protection space needs to be urgently addressed. Supervision, professional development, peer mentoring as well as manageable workload are urgently required for staff working with women with SUDs and their children.

Future directions

1. While early modelling of peer models for women and mothers with SUDs hold some hope, the sustainability and long term outcomes are not yet known. Therefore, peer models in SUDs should be further explored and trialled for women to ascertain if this has the potential to improve outcomes for women and their children, while protecting the trauma experienced by both peers and women.

2. Novel programs such as the PAUSE program from the UK should be examined for their feasibility and potentially piloted in the Australian context. An expansion of the FDTC into NSW is recommended.

3. A best practice guideline for women with children removed into OOHC is urgently needed.

Conclusion

This is the first known study in Australia that examines the needs and experiences of women in the perinatal period who are current injecting drug users. Finding indicate these women have multiple unmet health and psychosocial needs. Women had hoped to parent their children and had strong beliefs in their ability to do so, given the opportunity. The complexities within these women's lives including IPV, mental health, trauma, substance use meant that this was difficult to achieve at times. Additionally, women interacted with systems that hold power over them, fail to recognise their strengths and for some women basic needs such as housing were not met. Despite this, women valued positive relationships with professionals and the relational aspects of care were important to women's outcomes.

Care providers, including DCJ workers were passionate and dedicated professionals who wanted to make a difference to the lives of these women. However, these efforts were hampered through fragmented systems that do not adequately provide basic needs such as suitable housing, access to timely treatment and systems that stigmatise women and the workforce who provide care to them. A trial of models of care that proactively targets women with SUDs in their pregnancy and beyond such as nurse-led models of care and the proposed SHVP are urgently required. Pregnancy presents a unique window of opportunity for women with SUDs and they must be provided with accessible and acceptable care that harnesses women's strengths and presents ongoing opportunity for sustained change, beyond the perinatal period. Change is possible but committed action at all levels of the socioecological model is essential in order to break the cycle of adversity experienced by women and their children. Not doing so risks further and future generations of women and their children marred by SUDs, trauma, violence and generations of children living in OOHC. After all, and despite the challenges women face they, desired stability and normality, demonstrated by one final quote 'I want to have a family home, that's what I want in the end… if there were services … we could be supported as a family unit, then that would be perfect'.